Nikki Goldstein

Menopause The facts The fixes And The New you

Your Take-The-Power-Back Guide to Weight Loss
Hot Flashes and Loving Yourself Throughout "The Change"

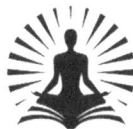

Go2Guru
PUBLISHING

ISBN   Hardcover: 978-1-923162-07-5
        Paperback: 978-1-923162-04-4
        E-Book: 978-1-923162-05-1

Cover design by Tika Design

Interior Formatting by 100Covers

Publisher: Go2Guru Publishing
www.go2gurupublishing.com

Disclaimer

Menopause The Facts The Fixes And The New You © 2023

Contents

Introduction

Nikki's Story

MY MOTHER ALWAYS carried a fan in her handbag. While there is something elegant, mysterious, and even sophisticated about the sight of a woman genteelly fanning her face, my mother regularly fanned herself as though trying to extinguish a fire. She'd pull up all her hair, which was drenched at the nape of her neck by the time the hot flash was upon her, collecting in dripping clumps, and furiously fan the back of her head. Rivers of perspiration would also gather on her forehead and run rudely down the sides of her face, gathering makeup as they rolled down her cheeks – which were suddenly flushed and red hot as though she'd just run a marathon. She'd start huffing and puffing and often say loudly, "Is it hot in here? Or is it just me?"

When Mom was in this state, we'd all duck for cover. The flash didn't just consume her body; it made her furious. For months, perhaps even years, the household was on eggshells. Mom was not herself. Little domestic issues, such as whose turn it was to do the dishes that night, turned into explosive rows with Mom raging at the center of the storm. My dad, a charming, charismatic but inveterate coward, hid at work and somehow managed to evade and ignore the changes that were happening to my mother. But with Dad often out of the line of sight, it left my siblings and me to deal with Mom's erratic moods and physical changes.

When I was about 14 and going through my own hormonal trials, I took my mother aside and said, "Mom, do you realize how hard you are to live with?" My mother was taken aback but admitted she felt out of control. An ex-nurse, Mom was quick to own up to the fact that even though she wasn't fully aware of how difficult she was to live with, she felt completely at the mercy of her menopausal symptoms. She hated the fact that she was putting on weight, even though her diet hadn't changed; she wasn't sleeping well, she felt crazy and angry all the time, and her relationship with my father was seemingly going off the rails.

That conversation with my mom happened more than 40 years ago. My mother didn't have access to the kinds of information, support and, importantly, the medical and alternative interventions that are available today. She went onto HRT in the early 1990s, which, she says, greatly helped balance her moods, but she went off it in the early 2000s when the breast cancer scare of the Women's Health Initiative report was released. Although it didn't kill her, my grandmother had had breast cancer, and Mom was advised, like millions of women all over the world, that the risks of breast cancer outweighed the benefits of HRT.

Despite the vast resources available to me as a long-time health and beauty journalist, my own menopause took me by surprise. Mom went into instant menopause at 50 because she had a hysterectomy. For some misguided reason, I thought I'd be spared the debilitating symptoms of menopause. How optimistic or deluded we can be!

Unlike my mom's surgery-induced menopause, my womb and ovaries were still happily residing in my body, but at exactly 50 years of age I started getting a raft of awful symptoms. It started with hot flashes. As part of my job reporting on beauty products, I was at a fancy function in a posh restaurant in the city. I was minding my own business when suddenly I felt like I was coming down with something. My head was swimming; I was confused. I felt hot and chilled all over, and my hands and fingers tingled. I thought I was having a stroke. A colleague at the table registered my discomfort and asked if I was OK. I ran to the bathroom in a panic. I wasn't just hot and bothered; I was burning up. Embarrassingly, my white t-shirt had turned grey under the armpits and at the back around my bra line. I stood awkwardly, my back bent pretzel-style, under a hand dryer, hoping to dry the telltale stains. I felt exposed and humiliated.

I returned to the table, but I couldn't regain my composure. I made an excuse that I had a headache and ran out of the restaurant as fast as my legs could carry me. But hot flashes were the tip of the iceberg. Soon, my sleep was interrupted by night sweats. I'd find myself jerking awake bathed in sweat, and my heart, generally a soft thrum in my veins, pulsing like a beating drum. In this condition, it was impossible to get back to sleep, and before long I had such terrible insomnia that I booked in to see the doctor.

I told the doctor I couldn't sleep, and I was walking around like a zombie. I had this strange, out-of-body sensation most days and brain fog. I told her that sometimes I'd forget my keys, wallet, or phone and that I was behaving erratically (the day before, I'd literally left a full shopping cart in the supermarket because I was so overcome by a hot flash that I couldn't wait in a queue to pay with my head roiling and sweat pouring down my back).

At that stage, I was still having periods, though scanty and irregular, and my doctor told me I was perimenopausal. From there, I went onto HRT, and I'm sure it saved my sanity, friendships, and marriage.

This book is not an exhortation for all women to use HRT. I'm not a doctor, and I'm not claiming that HRT is the be-all-and-end-all drug for all women. What I am saying is that if I was taken by surprise by menopause, when I had every bit of information at my fingertips, what does that mean for the many women in our world who don't have that access and feel at the mercy of their bodies?

Even Oprah, arguably one of the most powerful women in the world, with every advantage money and power can bring, was misdiagnosed before eventually being prescribed HRT for palpitations that doctors initially thought were heart disease. Since then, Oprah has broken many of the taboos about menopause and is still working to dispel the myths and misinformation surrounding this change of life.

I'm going to tell you a story about my friend Caro. Caro worked for a big advertising agency where most of her colleagues were men. One day, she felt a surge of wetness between her legs and, to her horror, looked down and saw a bright red bloom between her legs that was staining her beige skirt. She knew her period was due, but she'd never been caught out like that with so much blood. She grabbed her bag and ran to the lady's toilet, which happened not to be on her floor. So alarmed and embarrassed by the bright blood staining her skirt, she raced for the stairwell instead of taking the elevator (I wonder how many workplaces lack proper facilities close by for women?). Anyhow, by the time she'd navigated several flights of stairs and arrived at the restroom, so much blood had run down her legs that her ballet flats resembled a crimson Jackson Pollock. She said, "It looked like I'd been shot." Caro knew it had something to do with menopause, but she'd never heard of menorrhagia, the technical term for excessive menstrual bleeding associated with menopause.

Though it is rare to experience such excessive bleeding, Caro's doctor explained that one study found that among women aged between 42 - and 52, more than 90 percent experienced periods that lasted 10 days or more, with 78 percent reporting their flow as heavy.

Caro was mortified by what happened to her at work. And it wasn't the only time she experienced menorrhagia – it happened a few more times before she sought help from a specialist.

With all this gore and sweat and embarrassment, it's perhaps not surprising that menopause has been shrouded in secrecy. However, it's not merely the physical and psychological manifestations that have ensured there's a conspiracy of silence surrounding menopause – menopause has been stigmatized, stereotyped, and used as a political weapon against women for hundreds, if not thousands, of years.

My own pet theory is that shaming menopausal women takes away their power at precisely the moment in time when they're most likely to wield it.

Freed from our sexual marketability as a "maiden," liberated from our duties and responsibilities as a "mother," menopause marks the moment when we are truly free to be ourselves. It's a signal from nature that we can no longer conceive, and it's time for us to be prepared to embrace our wise woman "crone" archetype. Make no mistake, by the time menopause hits, most women are ready, willing, and able to accept themselves and the hotter and more bothered they become, the less willing they are to take any shit! Don't mess with a menopausal woman.

For too long, we've collectively bought into this idea that a woman is only valuable for her fertility and her beauty, and that older women are useless and worthless. This couldn't be further from the truth.

Witness women like Deborah Kilpatrick, the 55-year-old co-CEO and executive chair of Evidation Health, a digital health company worth $1 billion, who says that age "not only gives me more proverbial problem-solving arrows in my quiver, but it also allows me to more effectively use my energy." Sheila Johnson is not just the 74-year-old cofounder of BET Networks and Salamander Hotels and Resorts; she's also the first Black woman to own a stake in three sports franchises (the Washington Wizards, Capitals, and Mystics). Or look at Hoda Kotb, the 59-year-old TODAY Show co-anchor, who was 53 in 2018 when she scored the job. These women have not been cowed by being elders; they've actually turned the tables and used their years to enhance their power and position.

Even if we're not scaling the giddy heights of business, entertainment, or the arts, we've got much more power than we think. According to Forbes magazine, women over 50 have $15 trillion US dollars at their disposal. They represent 27 percent of all consumer spending and are responsible for 80 percent of all luxury purchases. Woefully, 91 percent of Boomer women feel ignored and misunderstood by marketers, yet 87 percent of Boomers and 90 percent of Gen X women are confident in using their incomes to fulfill their wishes (you're probably a Gen Xer if you're reading this – born between 1965 and 1981. Forbes reports that these groups of women will invest heavily in brands that align with their personal values.

In terms of an army of menopausal women covering the planet, according to the North American Menopause Society, by the year 2025, the number of postmenopausal women is expected to rise to 1.1 billion worldwide – which works out at about one-eighth of the total population. The United States alone had 50 million women over the age of 51 in 2020, and over two million U.S. women enter menopause annually. As populations all over the world age, these figures will only increase in the decades to come.

I say woe betide any government, institution, or company that neglects pre-menopausal, menopausal and post-menopausal women because we will be a purchasing and political force to be reckoned with! Not a threat but a reality.

Thankfully, in our time, the narrative is slowly changing and a small but growing battalion of impassioned scientists, doctors, and educators are helping to illuminate women about the issues around menopause and arming them with facts, not fiction.

As a journalist, my job is to do the legwork for you. This book brings together the most up-to-date science so you can be informed about the changes in your body – thereby empowering you to make the right decisions for you and your life. The book isn't a feminist rallying cry, but it is a shot over the bow to all the snake oil salespeople who aim to profit from our fears and insecurities. There is an industry around menopause, one that treats it as a disease to be cured rather than a stage of life to be managed and embraced.

The book's title, "Menopause: The Facts, The Fixes, And The New You," should hint at what I'm aiming to accomplish – to provide you with a handbook on how to thrive during this change of life. I wanted to dive into all the corners of a woman's life, from sex and sleep to style, and from hot flashes and mood swings to the profound spiritual and emotional changes we go through at this time of life. Most importantly, I wanted to arm you with information so you can drive these important conversations with your healthcare providers and empower yourself with the knowledge you need to make any changes necessary to live your best life.

For myself, I found HRT enormously helpful in the early stages of menopause; it literally restored me to myself. However, now that I'm through the swings and roundabouts of perimenopause, I've resorted to lifestyle changes to keep my mind, body, and spirit in balance. I use intermittent fasting and a diet brimming with Mediterranean-style nutrients to keep my weight in check. I have an exercise physiologist who works with me on strength, conditioning, and cardio (and by cardio, I really mean walking at a faster pace than a stroll). I have a team of other experts I rely on for my mental and spiritual well-being – a wonderful, insightful Jungian analyst, and an extraordinary hypnotherapist for the stuff I can't unearth on my own.

My background as a magazine and newspaper journalist has certainly aided me in my quest for information and understanding, but as I said, this book is the result of many years of research and trial and error. And just as a caveat, it's my choice to pay for the expert services of a highly qualified team to help me manage my health and wellbeing (and I forego other things in order to pay for these services – it's a priority and a choice I make on a daily and yearly basis). That said, this book is the result of the advice I've received from my team, and you'll benefit tremendously if you put in the work to accomplish your mind, body, and spirit goals as outlined in this book.

If you're at the stage where you're desperate to peel off your clothes all day, every day, wondering how to deal with the damned hot flashes, how to get rid of brain fog, or how to shed those pesky midline pounds, then this book is for you. I invite you to go on this journey with an open mind, ready to be challenged, inspired, informed, and empowered to enter this next chapter of your life as the heroine of your own story.

My mother recently said to me that I was lucky to live in this age. "You've got power because you've got information, and information gives you choices," she said. She's a wise old owl, my mom, and one who, despite the challenges of her times, has made the most of her life and her opportunities, though they were limited compared to mine. She inspires me to do my best every day.

Final Note: This book benefitted from the wise guidance of a brilliant physician who gave her time and expertise in crafting this work. I thank her from the bottom of my heart.

Nikki Goldstein

Part I

The Facts - A New Beginning - Reframe Your Mindset, Demystify Menopause, And Begin Anew With The Confidence Knowledge Brings

---

It's time to reset your body and mind with cutting-edge scientific and medical information to demystify, de-babble-ize, and educate yourself about menopause and its physical and psychological effects. You'll discover actionable advice that targets the very core of menopausal symptoms – your changing hormones. Information is power, so once you've learned the facts and jettisoned the fiction, you can embark on a journey of self-discovery and empowerment.

Chapter 1

Say Hello To Menopause

A FEW YEARS back, a woman sat in a restaurant in Copenhagen, the capital of Denmark. It was a Christmas market treat with some friends. Halfway through the meal, she felt discomfort in her lower body. Discomfort, which moments later, would feel like a volcano erupting in her nether regions. She went pale. She was cold in the seat as the warmth of liquid hit her legs.

This was Catherine O'Keeffe, educator, author, and founder of Wellness Warrior.

She sat still for what seemed like an eternity, frozen in fear. Eventually, she had the courage to put her head under the table. She was met with a deluge of blood that had soaked not only her but the wooden bench she was sitting on.

Hello, perimenopause!

On a freezing November night, she left that restaurant with her jacket around her waist and her head hanging with embarrassment. Little did she know at the time, gone were the days of wearing white trousers (for a while).

But for some reason, she decided she would fight it.

She was only 44. She wasn't ready for this!

Of course, perimenopause had other ideas.

Some weeks later, she was presenting to visiting management from New York. As a director in investment banking, she was used to meetings and presentations. In the room were two visiting executives, five of her own management team, herself, and one other uninvited, unexpected, and soon-to-arrive guest.

Menopause.

Just moments into her presentation, every piece of information she was hoping to present that day flew out of her head. Cue brain fog, memory loss, shame, anxiety – a menopause car crash. Her stomach sank, and she felt crucifying shame in front of her peers ... thankfully her manager saved her.

But menopause was here to stay.

Just like Catherine, most of us are underprepared and often resistant to the idea of menopause because it's been perceived as a taboo, something to hide and not talk about. But it's time for us to change this conversation.

Menopause is like this secret club no one really prepares you for. There's no question you'll be initiated into this club, but no one tells you what hoops you'll have to jump through. The only thing you probably know is that one day, your ovaries will stop producing eggs, and you won't have your period anymore.

But guess what? It's not the endgame – it's the start of a whole new level. To quote Dr. Maureen Gaffney, "We have to go back in order to go forwards. Because change is difficult."

Change is hard. And menopause is *the* change.

Imagine it as a plot twist in your life story—a chance to grab a pen and write a whole new chapter. You're not fading into the background; you're taking center stage. In this chapter, we're flipping the script on menopause. Because this isn't a decline; it's a makeover.

Most of us have been conditioned to view this as the end. Period. No coming back from the death of your fertility, right?

Wrong.

Let me break it down for you. This natural biological process as part of your body's clock has not rung its final bell just yet.

Does menopause mean your monthly monster will no longer visit you?

Why, yes, it does.

Does it mean you will no longer be able to have children?

Yes, it does.

But does it mean your life is over or you will never have any joy again?

Most definitely not!

Catherine O'Keeffe believed so strongly that the topic of menopause was a conversation we should all be having that she quit her investment banking job and created Wellness Warrior, a coaching service for corporations grappling with the issues menopause brings up in the workplace. She says, "Menopause offers the opportunity to look at where you're at in life and assess and prepare for the years ahead."

Menopause is a journey of discovery and self-realization. It's a time to embrace, not fight, the changes that are taking place in your body and to learn how to make the most of life's second half. This is a time to rise up and take your power back – from the institutions that seek to put women out to pasture (at a certain age), from the misogyny we find in our communities and the media, and even from the relationships that may want to pigeon-hole us as past our prime. When we own our power as mature women, nothing can stop us!

Embracing The Mid-Life Rebirth

The inescapable truth of life is that at some point, our bodies will no longer be the same, and we have to accept the fact that our lives are changing. Think of it this way: not all women will become pregnant or give birth, but every woman, if she lives long enough, will go through menopause.

We're all headed there at some point or other. So, why are we so scared to talk about it?

Because it's often associated with being "old" and the loss of youth and attractiveness, there's a lot of mystery, misinformation, misogyny, and confusion surrounding menopause – and for a good reason.

Since the dawn of time, the only record we have about this major transition has been written primarily by men. Can you imagine how they bungled it? Let's start in the Middle Ages when male physicians deemed menopause a "nervous disorder" where a woman ceased to exist as a sexual being. Humoural Theory posited that when menstruation finished that a woman became tainted, polluted, and a threat to the natural order. Commonly, menopausal women were cast out of society and called witches (and we know how that worked out for women thought to be engaged in witchcraft).

Fast forward to the nineteenth century, when menopausal symptoms were often blamed on a life of idleness. At the same time, Sir Edward Tilt penned the first comprehensive book on menopause. He classified menopause as a condition encompassing 137 varied symptoms. Not bad. Menopause does cause a wide variety of symptoms. Some interesting examples he mentioned include "pseudo-narcolepsy," "temporary deafness," and "uncontrollable peevishness." And let's not forget my personal favorite – brace yourself – "hysterical flatulence."

But to be fair, the average lifespan worldwide at that time was 33 years old, and in Europe, it was just 43 years old. So, the majority of menopausal women were already dead.

You would think by 1900, men would have come up with something better than "hysterical flatulence." But no. It was only in the 1970s that women started to gain control over their own medical narratives. The pioneering work of Dr. Robert Wilson catalyzed this shift by emphasizing the natural aspects of menopause and making it a part of a woman's overall health narrative rather than an illness.

But even then, his book boldly stated, "The unpalatable truth must be faced that all postmenopausal women are cast stray."

Unpalatable? Cast stray?

You can see how menopause used to be seen as the bringer of death based on those records. However, Wilson didn't leave menopausal women to face their bleak destiny. Instead, a pharmaceutical solution was proposed: estrogen replacement therapy (ERT). He argued that ERT, like insulin, had the potential to cure and prevent estrogen deficiency disease. By preserving women's sexual vitality, long-term hormone therapy averted the "greatest tragedy" in women's lives.

Thanks to advancements in medical technology and greater numbers of women taking on roles as physicians, doctors were able to diagnose and treat menopause more professionally and with less bias. In the 80s and 90s, women's health became a hot topic, with organizations like The North American Menopause Society (NAMS) forming in '89.

In 1992, Gail Sheehy released her groundbreaking book "The Silent Passage," which shined a light on menopause and its effects. She boldly wrote about her own experience and brought menopause out of the shadows.

Also, during the 1990s, research was being conducted to determine how hormone therapy could prevent disease during postmenopausal life. The Women's Health Initiative (WHI) launched in 1993, with 15,000 women participating. The WHI hormone studies had the goal of checking if hormone treatment could prevent heart disease, fractures, and mental deterioration as women age. They mainly relied on info from women who started hormone therapy around menopause and continued it in an observational way. To really understand the effects, WHI wanted to do a clinical trial and see the benefits, especially in older women with more risk factors.

But panic ensued when they shut it down in 2002, and the message that women got was:

Hormones are no good!

Hormones are going to give you breast cancer!

Hormones are going to give you a heart attack!

Hormones are going to give you a stroke!

The headlines that came out of this study set women back half a century or so. Women were catapulted back to the pre-HRT era – where you had to suffer in silence and live with your symptoms.

Although it was later explained that for younger women the risk is minimal, and the potential benefits of HRT can be substantial, unfortunately, despite subsequent analyses not showing significant risk of breast cancer, this initial impression deeply impacted women's perceptions for over 20 years.

Women lost years just because of one study. They felt betrayed, and still, to this day, there is a lack of trust among women with regard to HRT.

The good news is we are now in a place where more accurate information is available, where menopause is much less of a taboo subject, and women are more empowered to take control of their health. They are increasingly more likely to do their own research and make decisions for themselves. Thank heavens for the internet!

In part, this book is about putting a guide into your hands so you can make important decisions about your body yourself. Power springs from education and information. The misinformation the Women's Health

Initiative conveyed dissuaded and prevented women from getting the help they needed for a generation. I don't want that to happen again!

So, let's take a deep dive into what menopause is and what leads up to it.

Perimenopause Vs. Menopause

Just as we saw in Catherine's story, the end can begin with a bang, not a whimper. If you were someone who had the most regular periods, and suddenly that predictable schedule vanished – that's a sign you might be in perimenopause.

On average, perimenopause can start up to a decade before menopause. During this phase, your body will begin to produce fewer and lower levels of hormones. Estrogen levels fluctuate significantly, often declining but with occasional spikes. Progesterone levels may also decrease gradually. These hormonal shifts impact the menstrual cycle regularity, causing changes in flow and frequency of periods. Other hormones like testosterone and follicle-stimulating hormone (FSH) might also fluctuate, contributing to various symptoms like hot flashes, mood swings, sleep disturbances, low libido, headaches, sore breasts, weight gain, and vaginal dryness just to name a few..

For some, perimenopause lasts a few months, while for others, it can last four to eight years – navigating this period can be challenging. It's a time when you may need coping strategies and support to get through it.

Conversely, menopause itself is clocked from a specific day – when you haven't experienced any menstrual bleeding for 12 consecutive months. While it might not be easy to pinpoint that exact day, it's the milestone that defines menopause. The average age for menopause in the United States is 51, but it can range from 40-60, so it's best to be prepared for the changes that come with it.

Estrogen and progesterone levels drop significantly and stabilize at lower levels consistently. The absence of these hormones at their usual levels affects various body systems, leading to symptoms like vaginal dryness, hot flashes, mood changes, and bone density loss.

Why Understanding Menopause Matters

Because each of us is a distinct, unique individual, you will not have the same menopause as your sister, your cousin, your neighbor, or any other woman in the world.

Our experiences with perimenopause and menopause are going to be vastly different from woman to woman. The age at which we go through the severity of our symptoms – which organ systems it's affecting the most – will change. This is where we should exercise caution and not use our own experience to judge or even try to educate other women (and leave that to the professionals) because no two women will experience menopause in the same way.

It's a fallacy that menopause is some generic condition, like a cold. At this time of significant physical and emotional change, it's worth remembering that we could be kinder and more understanding towards each other – but most particularly to ourselves.

Unfortunately, there is not a single, simple test to determine when a woman begins perimenopause. Nope. No testing is available. So, you and your healthcare provider must do some investigative work. And this is where a lot of healthcare providers are undertrained or under-utilizing the resources available to them.

Everybody wants easy, including healthcare providers; they want a quick test, something super no-fuss. But, because of the massive fluctuations in our hormone levels during perimenopause, we do not have a good, reliable test that will consistently tell you if you're perimenopausal 100 percent of the time.

But how would you know if you are finally at that stage?

There are actually so many symptoms of perimenopause that sometimes you don't even remember which ones to talk about and which ones to let go. However, there are self-assessment tools and symptom checkers available online that can help. And guess what? Qualified healthcare professionals can even administer a few assessment tools clinically. These include:

- Menopause Specific Quality of Life Questionnaire (MENQOL) – designed to assess the health and quality of life of menopausal women.
- Kupperman Index – a standardized assessment tool to measure hot flashes, night sweats, and other perimenopause symptoms.
- Menopause Rating Scale (MRS) – a 15-item assessment tool to determine menopausal and perimenopausal symptom severity.

As a starting point, we've added two quick, easy, interactive quizzes (the first at the end of this chapter, and the second one at the back of this book), as well as an extensive symptom checker so you can tick off your symptoms. It's by no means a medical diagnosis, but it's designed to be a conversation starter between you and your physician. You may be surprised by some of the less common symptoms that you might have overlooked.

Using the medical assessments and guides such as the ones included here, you'll kickstart your menopause journey. I highly recommend using a journal or tracker. Your healthcare providers will benefit from understanding the evolution of menopause symptoms over time, including variations in intensity and occurrence patterns. A symptom diary (you can do this either on paper or digitally using apps like Clue, Ovia, and Flo) will give you powerful and valuable data. When noting your symptoms, pay attention to where they originate from – brain fog, physical fatigue, or joint pain. Whether to use these apps or go old school with a pen and paper is totally your call. Either way works just fine!

Jessica, a 43-year-old mom of two, used a symptom diary to keep track of her perimenopausal symptoms. She found that by writing down when she experienced headaches, hot flashes, mood swings, and other issues, she was able to understand better how these symptoms were impacting her life – and plan for the future. But she also said, "Journaling saved my sanity. I thought I was losing it! It helped me understand the true impact of my symptoms, and I was able to make better decisions as a result."

When tracking symptoms, note the date, time, associated factors, location, intensity, and duration. Also, observe if symptoms improve or worsen and what provides relief. Include any relevant measures taken, like medications or treatments. This log helps you and your doctor understand the underlying cause or condition, considering both the symptoms and their impact on your life.

For menopause, there are several tests you can consider. Some you can do at home, or go to a clinic for procedures like ultrasound or a blood test. However, the most accurate test is a hormone panel that measures FSH and estradiol levels. This type of test provides a detailed picture of any hormonal imbalances you might be experiencing. You can gain valuable insights into your body's condition by checking your estrogen, testosterone, progesterone, and DHEA-S levels.

The clinical diagnosis is important for tracking your progress and getting the best advice from your doctor. But perhaps more importantly, in the battle against misinformation and in the name of self-empowerment, it's vital to understand the storm that's raging inside you. Women deserve to know what's happening inside their bodies, and a diagnosis is a critical claim on territory often ignored by the medical establishment.

Never forget: You are your own best advocate. Never be afraid to ask for more tests, or change physicians if you don't feel your issues are being adequately addressed or you feel dismissed or derided. When it comes to your body, you are in the driver's seat; you have the power to walk away from any situation that makes you feel uncomfortable or unheard. Be proactive and take the power back.

Finally, a proper diagnosis will also help you get a grip on the mental changes you may be experiencing. There's no doubt one of the casualties of this tsunami is your mind.

Mood Swings, Mental Mayhem And Menopause

Marina Gask, a well-known journalist and editor from South London, went through some tough times with her family due to the challenges of menopause.

Even the most minor things her husband and two teenage sons did triggered feelings of intense anger. And it wasn't their fault – she couldn't control those emotions. "They were probably just being their usual (sometimes thoughtless) selves, but I constantly felt hurt and full of irrational anger. Why didn't they understand how I was feeling? Why didn't they seem to care?" she said. When Marina started experiencing symptoms like irregular periods, frequent overheating, and skin irritations at 48, she became anxious but couldn't articulate why.

It was tough for Marina to talk about menopause with her sons because she had always been the strong "Mom" figure who didn't show her emotions. She was scared and embarrassed, and that kept her from opening up, resulting in breakdowns and irrational behavior.

And she is not the only one.

Up to 70 percent of women experience irritability during menopause. Mood changes like anger and rage can impact your menopause journey, starting from the earliest signs of perimenopause all the way to post-menopause.

During perimenopause, the changes in hormones that impact your periods can also mess with your emotions. As if that wasn't enough, dealing with weight gain, insomnia, and burning as hot as a furnace can pile on stress and fatigue, making everything seem like the end of the world.

Your 40s and 50s are already the time when life's pressures tend to hit the hardest.

It's a lot to juggle balancing demanding jobs, taking care of young kids or sending older ones off to college, and looking after aging parents. All of this stress can really take a toll on your mental health.

You would think because you are no longer having your period, you might be given a reprieve from the dreaded PMS. Unfortunately, perimenopausal symptoms can be just as intense, if not more so, than those you experienced during your reproductive years.

About four in ten women experience mood symptoms during perimenopause that can be similar to PMS, or premenstrual syndrome. You might feel irritable, have low energy, be teary and moody, or have trouble focusing. The interesting thing is, unlike PMS, these symptoms can happen at any time, not just during your menstrual cycle. And here's the crazy part – these symptoms can go on for years without any pattern.

It's called perimenopausal mood instability.

Depression, anxiety, and panic attacks can also be part of it. It's a real puzzle to figure out and often requires trial and error to find the proper treatment. In some cases, lifestyle changes may be enough. But for others, hormone therapy, antidepressants, or other medication might help.

For those already dealing with mental health issues, these changes can make things more complicated. Some medications for mental health can also affect how our bodies handle these changes.

When mental health and menopause intersect, it can affect not just how we feel but also our overall physical health in the long run. To navigate this journey better, doctors and mental health professionals need to work together.

Sometimes, this might involve making lifestyle changes or considering hormone therapy. The good news is there are lots of options available for managing these symptoms. Talk to your doctor or a mental health professional to figure out what might work best for you. And remember, you don't have to go through it alone – plenty of resources and support are available. With the right combination of treatments and care, you can get back on track and feel like yourself again.

Marina found relief with acupuncture, and by 52, her periods and all the symptoms stopped forever. By 60, she'd implemented a raft of lifestyle changes like regular running, and also found how important honesty was in her relationship with her husband and sons.

I can't stress enough how important it is to talk about mental health and the struggles associated with it. Even if you don't have a pre-diagnosed mental illness, menopause can disrupt your psychological equilibrium. In this circumstance, the most empowered thing you can do is seek professional advice.

Now that you've armed yourself with essential knowledge and practical tools for understanding and diagnosing menopause and the mental turmoil that often goes hand in hand with this transition, let's tackle another crucial aspect: hormones. Chapter 2 will help you understand how these invisible chemicals shape your menopause experience and how you can manage them effectively.

Before you move onto Chapter 2, fill out this easy and interactive quiz. It's designed to help you get a snapshot of where you're at on your menopause journey. It's not a stand-in for a consultation with your doctor, but it will help you figure out where you're at while you read through this book.

Menopause Symptom Quiz #1

Section 1: Physical Symptoms

1. Hot Flashes
   - Have you experienced sudden, intense feelings of heat, sometimes accompanied by flushing and sweating?

2. Night Sweats
   - Do you often wake up drenched in sweat during the night, leading to disrupted sleep patterns?

3. Irregular Periods
   - Have your menstrual cycles become irregular or stopped altogether?

4. Vaginal Changes
   - Have you noticed dryness, itching, burning, or discomfort in the vaginal area, especially during sexual intercourse?

5. Sleep Disturbances
   - Have you had difficulties falling asleep or staying asleep?

6. Changes in Body Composition
   - Have you experienced weight gain, particularly around the abdomen, or changes in body shape that are hard to explain through diet or exercise?

7. Physical Sensitivity
- Have you noticed increased joint pain, muscle aches, or general physical discomfort without an obvious cause?

Section 2: Emotional and Mental Health Symptoms

8. Mood Swings
- Do you find yourself experiencing mood swings, feeling irritable, anxious, or having sudden emotional shifts?

9. Memory Issues
- Have you experienced memory lapses, forgetfulness, or difficulty concentrating?

10. Changes in Libido
- Have you noticed a decrease in your interest or desire for sexual activity?

11. Emotional Health
- Have you felt an overall change in your emotional well-being, experiencing feelings of sadness, depression, or a lack of motivation?

Section 3: Physical Changes

12. Skin and Hair Changes
- Have you noticed changes in your skin such as dryness, increased wrinkling, or changes in hair texture or thickness?

13. Cardiovascular Changes
- Have you experienced palpitations, changes in heart rate, or fluctuations in blood pressure?

14. Digestive Issues
- Have you had more digestive problems like bloating, gas, or changes in bowel habits since the onset of menopause symptoms?

Scoring

Give yourself 1 point for each "Yes" answer.
- 0-4 points: Low likelihood of menopausal symptoms.
- 5-9 points: Moderate likelihood of experiencing menopausal symptoms.
- 10-14 points: Higher likelihood of menopausal symptoms.

This assessment is not a substitute for professional medical advice. If you suspect you're experiencing menopausal symptoms, consult with a healthcare provider for accurate evaluation and appropriate guidance.

Chapter 2

Demystifying The Hormone Changes

WHEN ELLA HIT 38, her life took an unexpected turn, and her once-steady rhythm became a whirlwind of uncertainty and unexplained emotions. Mood swings and random bouts of sadness took over, overshadowing the vibrant life she once had.

She started by seeing a general physician in hopes of finding relief from her overwhelming symptoms. She got some tests done to check for thyroid issues and hormonal imbalances. Not finding anything, her doctor gave her antidepressants. She said, "It felt like applying sticky tape to stop a leak in a dam."

After some discussions with her friends, Ella went on a quest for answers. She was young; no way would she be going through menopause. However, after doing some research online, she found that the physical and emotional symptoms she was experiencing were quite typical for women her age.

As it turns out, Ella's hormones had gone haywire, a condition known as perimenopause. So, she sought out a menopause specialist who recognized the importance of hormone replacement therapy (HRT) in restoring balance and prescribed an HRT plan tailor-made for Ella.

The change was remarkable. Within weeks of starting HRT, Ella noticed a big shift. The chaos started to resolve. The hot flashes became more bearable, the sadness lifted, and the mood swings settled.

It wasn't just a change in symptoms but a real return to herself.

Ella's story might resonate with you. How many times do you think women get misdiagnosed with a mental illness when the real problem is something else entirely?

The answer is more than you think. Hormone deficiencies are extremely common in women experiencing perimenopause, but it's often misdiagnosed as depression or anxiety. The question is, how do you get the right treatment?

To answer that question, you first need to understand your body's delicate dance of hormones.

The Science Behind The Hormonal Symphony

As a Chinese proverb wisely states, "A wise (wo)man adapts himself to circumstances, as water shapes itself to the vessel that contains it." And while we are no longer the flexible twenty-year-olds who might be able to make like "water" and move fluidly through life, we can still learn to adapt and embrace "The Change."

Whether you're going through it or know someone who is, it's vital to recognize there's nothing to fear. Technically, "menopause" is diagnosed one year after the final period. But most people use it to refer to the entire span of time when our menstrual cycle is changing in length. As we discussed in the previous chapter, this process usually lasts several years.

So, it's best to think of menopause as a continuum starting years before, during what is called the menopause transition – or like puberty in reverse.

Just like puberty, the process takes place over many years. When we're born, we actually have all the eggs we're ever going to make (around one to two million of them), just chilling out in the ovaries in an immature state. When we hit around eight to ten years old, the hypothalamus, a part of our brain, starts releasing a hormone called gonadotropin-releasing hormone (GnRH). It basically says, "Hey eggs, wake up!" as luteinizing hormone (LH) and follicle-stimulating hormone (FSH) kick it into action.

And that's when the whole monthly ovulation thing happens.

This is what increases the production of a class of hormones you've probably heard about – estrogen. Estrogen and other hormones begin a delicate hormonal dance that, once a month, results in the most mature egg leaving its follicle and travelling down a fallopian tube. The body builds up the lining in the uterus, the endometrium, to house the egg, and if the egg isn't fertilized, the lining sheds.

And we are granted menstruation. The gift that keeps on giving!

Of course, that's just the overview of ovulation. It's a complex process regulated by your endocrine system with hormones like the aforementioned estrogen, LH, progesterone, FSH, human chorionic gonadotropin (hCG), inhibin, and more. All these hormones work in concert to ensure that the process goes smoothly, from the creation of a follicle to ovulation and menstruation.

This cycle repeats over and over and over for decades.

On average, sometime in the mid-forties, ovulation becomes erratic. We don't have as many eggs, and the ones that remain may not be as healthy as they once were. Estrogen can be lower in some cycles and higher during others. This is the menopause transition. Hormonal chaos – just like puberty. Only this time, when estrogen levels stabilize, they'll be much lower than they were before.

This very normal decrease in estrogen and other hormonal changes does come with medical concerns, such as osteoporosis, heart disease, diabetes, and vaginal dryness. Some of us are lucky and will have mild or no symptoms. Others will experience trouble sleeping, irritability, depression, or decreased sex drive.

And then there's the most classic symptom: hot flashes. They're a wave of heat that makes it feel like a furnace just got cranked up on the inside. Scientists aren't entirely sure why this happens, but the resulting heat makes you feel sweaty and off-kilter. Some women even have symptoms that overlap with anxiety, like nausea and palpitations. Let's look at how hormonal fluctuations cause typical symptoms of menopause.

Hot Flashes: 75 to 80 percent of menopausal women experience the furnace-like flush of hot flashes. Our bodies become overheated when our hypothalamus, a small region in the brain that regulates body temperature, mistakenly thinks we are too cold and triggers an increase in heat through vasodilation. This is why hot flashes can be accompanied by sweating.

Estrogen plays a significant role in regulating body temperature. As estrogen levels fluctuate during menopause, it can affect the hypothalamus. The hypothalamus might get confused and react as if the body is overheating, leading to sudden heat sensations, flushing, sweating, and sometimes palpitations.

Mood Swings: Estrogen and progesterone also influence neurotransmitters like serotonin and dopamine, which regulate mood. Fluctuations in these hormones during menopause can disrupt the balance of these neurotransmitters, potentially leading to mood swings, irritability, anxiety, or depression.

Weight Gain: Hormonal changes, particularly a decrease in estrogen, can affect metabolism and fat distribution. Lower estrogen levels may contribute to weight gain, especially around the abdomen. Additionally, hormonal shifts might affect appetite regulation and energy expenditure, making it easier to gain weight during menopause.

Bone Loss: Estrogen helps regulate calcium metabolism and bone remodeling activities. When estrogen levels drop during menopause, the balance between these two activities is disrupted, leading to increased bone loss. Not only can this lead to an increased risk of fracture, but it might also be linked to issues like osteoporosis or other bone-related diseases.

These symptoms vary in intensity and occurrence among individuals due to differences in hormonal fluctuations and other factors. Understanding these hormonal changes can help you make informed decisions about whether you need to make lifestyle changes or seek medical help.

HRT: Decoding The Menopausal Dilemma

Gabriela, a woman from Mexico in the prime of her life, faced unexpected challenges. At 38, her life seemed perfect: happily married with three children, a dog, and a demanding but rewarding job. However, after deciding to cease the contraceptive pill, her world turned upside down. Gabriela experienced diverse symptoms, including mood swings, low energy, irritability, and irregular periods. She sought opinions from multiple doctors and was finally diagnosed with post-menopause.

"Post-menopause, he said. Post? So, it was over? I'd gone through it all *a pelo*, like we say in Mexico: cold turkey. But once he started me on hormonal therapy, my life was transformed."

So, hormone therapy – what does it mean when we say hormone therapy, menopause hormone therapy, MHT, hormone replacement therapy, or HRT?

In layman's terms, it's about giving hormones back during the estrogen-deficient state associated with perimenopause and menopause. The main hormone we are talking about is estrogen. There are several ways to get this medication into your body.

Estrogen

In our bodies, there are three types of circulating estrogen. The primary one is *estradiol*, a highly bioactive estrogen produced in the ovaries that serves as the main component. *Estriol* is predominantly produced during pregnancy, with minimal presence otherwise. Lastly, *estrone* is synthesized by peripheral tissues, particularly fat cells, through androgens like testosterone.

Put simply, estradiol is the most bioactive of these hormones. Estriol really only comes into its own in pregnancy, and estrone is in varying levels depending on how much fat tissue you have and is not really considered to be that bioactive. You can have high levels of it, but it does not cause nearly the same effects as estradiol does when we are making decisions about hormone replacement therapy.

When discussing **synthetic** hormone replacement therapy, we typically refer to variations like ethinyl estradiol or norethindrone. Alternatively, we may mention conjugated equine estrogens, commonly known as Premarin. Which stands for pregnant mare urine because – you guessed it – it's derived from the urine of pregnant horses.

Types of HRT

HRT is available as tablets, patches, gels, or vaginal treatments. The type of HRT you need and the associated risks will vary according to:

- Your age
- Whether you have had a hysterectomy
- Whether you have other health conditions.

Your doctor can tailor the type of hormone treatment best suited to you. If you had an early menopause, the current recommendation is that you should continue treatment at least until the average age of menopause (51 years).

Estrogen + Progestogen

If you still have your uterus (have not had a hysterectomy), you need a treatment that combines estrogen and progestogen. Progestogens (including norethisterone, medroxyprogester, one dydrogesterone, and micronized progesterone) are added to the treatment to reduce the risk of cancer of the uterus. Here are the safety facts:

- Doesn't cause weight gain

- Blood clots – patches and gels have minimal or no risk. When using tablets, the risk doubles but is still very low (one extra case per 1,000 women).
- Heart disease – no increased risk if HRT begins within 10 years of onset of menopause or before the age of 60.
- Breast cancer – overall, one in eight women will develop breast cancer during their lifetime. The added risk of breast cancer with HRT is minimal. The risk increases the longer you take HRT and decreases after stopping. Using a different progestogen may reduce the risk.
- Stroke – no increased risk for women without underlying stroke risk factors who are in their 50s or during the first 10 years of menopause. Women with risk factors can probably safely use a patch or gel form of treatment.

Estrogen By Itself

Estrogen alone is suitable for women who have had a hysterectomy. Here are the safety facts:

- **Blood Clots:** Patches and gels have minimal or no risk. When using tablets, the risk doubles but is still very low (one extra case per 1000 women).
- **Heart Disease:** May decrease the risk of heart disease if started within 10 years of menopause or before the age of 60.
- **Breast Cancer:** Overall, one in eight women will develop breast cancer during their lifetime. Studies suggest that there is either no increase or a minimal added risk of breast cancer when using estrogen-only HRT. Breast cancer risk is lower with estrogen-only HRT compared with estrogen plus progestogen.
- **Stroke:** No increased risk for women without underlying stroke risk factors who are in their 50s or during the first 10 years of menopause. Women with risk factors can probably safely use a patch or gel form of treatment.

Vaginal Estrogen Therapy

Vaginal estrogen therapy is helpful for women who have local symptoms such as vaginal dryness. Here are the safety facts:

- Vaginal estrogen therapy is safe to use long-term – except after breast cancer.

SERMs

Selective estrogen receptor molecules (SERMs) are hormone therapies that manage how estrogen works in the body. SERMs such as tamoxifen and raloxifene, which you've probably heard of in relation to breast cancer, are also effective treatments for osteoporosis.

Think of them as medical multitaskers: for a start, they block estrogen from colliding with breast cancer cells and prevent them from multiplying. At the same time, they boost estrogen levels in your bones and help prevent osteoporosis.

Recently, SERMS has been recognized as a treatment option for menopause. They have both anti-estrogen and estrogen-like effects that vary in different parts of the body. A pill containing conjugate equine estrogen combined with the SERM bazedoxifene has been shown to improve menopausal symptoms and bone density and reduce breast density. In women who have not had a hysterectomy SERMs can reduce the risk of cancer of the lining of the uterus. As a treatment option speak to your doctor.

Bio-Identical Hormones: You might have heard celebrities and even girlfriends tout the benefits of bio-identical hormones. The claim is that they'll not only disappear menopause symptoms, but they'll also wind back the clock. It's true they're popular. Clinicians in the US estimate that between 26 to 33 million prescriptions for compounded bioidentical hormones (cBHT) are filled each year, and almost 41 percent of women who need treatment for menopausal symptoms have tried cBHT in their lives. However, both the North American Menopause Society and the US Preventative Services Task Force recommend against the use of non-FDA-approved therapies such as cBHT.

Before you take them, you should know that no study resolutely proves their efficacy. Here are some points to consider when making a decision:

Regulation And Consistency: The production of bio-identical hormones often occurs in compounding pharmacies, where formulations can vary widely in potency and consistency. These labs also don't adhere to FDA regulations often. When the FDA did secret shopper testing on the ten largest compounding labs that were making pellets in the USA, they found a 34 percent discrepancy between what they said was in the pellet and what was actually in the pellet. One 2021 study published in "Menopause" comparing patients on cBHT or FDA-approved HRT found that side effects were significantly higher in the cBHT group, at 57.6 percent, compared to the HRT group at just 14.8 percent. The Australasian Menopause Society goes so far as to say it does "not recommend the use of cBHT in any form including creams, lozenges and pessaries." It also says that the use of cBHT has been associated with endometrial cancer and that the marketing hype surrounding the notion that cBHT is more "natural" is spurious.

Safety Concerns: The safety profile of bio-identical hormones is not well-studied. While they might be structurally similar to natural hormones, their effects on health and long-term risks are not fully understood. Comprehensive research on bio-identical hormones is substantially lacking, and using them may increase the risk of side effects.

Personalized Dosing: Companies of bio-identical hormones claim these hormones can be tailored to meet individual needs. While that might sound tempting, the absence of standardized dosages makes it tough to figure out the right amount, which could result in imbalanced hormone levels and unwanted side effects.

Ultimately, the term "bio-identical hormones" might sound sexy, but it can also oversimplify a complex issue. While they might offer some benefits for some women, the lack of comprehensive scientific research and standardized production raises concerns about their safety and efficacy.

Your power as a consumer of health care products resides in your ability to decode the hype, do the research (which is what this book is all about), and get good, clear answers to your questions. Consulting a doctor for *personalized advice* and considering all available options is probably your best strategy before deciding on any treatment for menopausal symptoms.

Navigating The Facts (Not The Fiction) Of HRT

When it comes to hormone replacement therapy, oral estradiol is a cost-effective and body-identical option that comes with different strengths. However, it does carry a small risk of increased clotting factors, which means it may not be suitable for people at risk of **stroke**. This is something to discuss with your physician.

On the other hand, transdermal forms like patches, gels, and creams significantly lower the risk of blood clots. So, if you're advised against hormone replacement therapy due to clotting concerns, going for transdermal administration may be a good option.

Now, let's talk about progesterone. The synthetic progestins used in breast cancer studies have shown an increased risk of breast cancer. Let me be clear here: synthetic progesterone, called progestin, has been shown to increase the risk of breast cancer. Not natural progesterone!

Although we still don't know why synthetic hormones like progestins increase breast cancer risk, there is robust data that implies an association. A large study in France found that using estrogen and progesterone did not increase the risk of breast cancer, while using estrogen plus progestin increased the risk by 16-69 percent, depending on the type of progestin. Although the actual risk is relatively low, for example, women aged 16 to 20 who use hormonal contraceptives may experience eight additional cases of breast cancer per 100,000 users. This shifts perspective from percentage-based statistics.

But don't worry, there's a safer alternative – body-identical progesterone.

Unfortunately, transdermal options for body-identical progesterone are limited, so oral intake is necessary. However, many people combine an estrogen transdermal patch with an oral progesterone pill to get a fully body-identical approach.

One side effect that gained traction in the early days was the risk of *breast cancer* with combined therapy. While there's a slight increase in risk after about seven years of use, it's similar to some other medications or being obese. This elevated risk equates to about one in a thousand women. Surprisingly, women on hormone replacement therapy have a lower mortality rate from cancer compared to those not on HRT.

To further put your mind at ease, the North American Menopause Society's 2022 statement on hormone replacement therapy *concluded that for nearly all women under 60 without absolute contraindications, the benefits significantly outweigh the risks.*

When considering whether to take HRT, it's essential to discuss any absolute contraindications, like active liver or heart disease and specific breast cancer risks, with a healthcare provider.

In the end, if you decide not to go for hormone replacement therapy, it's totally up to you. But it's crucial to have a real talk with your doctor. Considering your unique health history and family history, the risks and benefits are all things you deserve to know.

When To Start HRT?

The idea that you have to wait until your blood shows specific things before treatment is simply not true! It's a misconception. You can start getting help for perimenopause whenever you need it. There are people who started HRT in their late 30s or 40s because it was necessary for them. So, it's all about what's right for you and your health – not some fake news story you found on Google.

Recent studies also suggest that starting hormone replacement therapy (HRT) early in menopause may lower the risk of Alzheimer's and dementia. However, if you wait until symptoms have already begun, it could potentially make things worse.

So, timing is key. When it comes to both cardiovascular disease and neurodegenerative conditions, starting HRT early, very early, seems to offer the most benefits. But if you wait too long, it might not have the same positive impact and provide the results you seek.

Natural Ways to Manage Menopause

It's true that not every woman wants or needs to take HRT. Natural alternatives do exist and include various dietary supplements, herbal remedies, and alternative therapies. However, it's essential to approach these alternatives with caution and consult a healthcare professional before adding them to your routine due to limited regulation and varying research supporting their effectiveness. Here are some options:

Dietary Supplements:

- B Vitamins: Help regulate energy and cell production, potentially reducing hot flashes.
- Vitamin E: Helps neutralize oxidative stress and might improve hot flashes.
- Vitamin D: Essential for bone health and may regulate hormones and vaginal dryness.
- Omega-3s: May aid in lubrication and, when taken with SSRIs, could improve depression.
- Resveratrol: A 2020 study showed 14-week supplementation with low-dose resveratrol improved blood flow in the brain and cognitive function and improved pain perception and quality of life.

NB: it's always better to supply your nutritional needs from food sources, but when dietary intake is inadequate, supplementation can assist with meeting your daily nutrient requirements.

Herbal Supplements:

- Black Cohosh: May help decrease hot flashes.
- St. John's Wort: Could improve sleep quality during and after menopause.
- Dong Quai: Acts similarly to estrogen, potentially balancing hormones.
- Chaste Tree: Might have hormone-balancing effects, impacting menopause symptoms.
- Maca: May assist in balancing hormones and improving sexual function.
- Red Clover: Contains isoflavones acting like estrogen, potentially relieving hot flashes.
- Sage: May minimize hot flashes and other menopause symptoms.
- Milk Thistle: Contains isoflavones that may help balance hormones and help prevent osteoporosis.
- Valerian Root and Hops: Herbal sleep aids that might reduce sleep disturbances.
- Evening Primrose Oil: High in fatty acids that may help with body lubrication.
- Ginseng, Licorice: Ginseng might boost mood, while licorice may help adrenal health and reduce hot flashes.
- Soy isoflavones or phytoestrogens: May help hot flashes, but do not take them if you can't take prescribed HRT.
- Wild yam cream: Has gained traction for its effectiveness in treating menopausal symptoms but there is no scientific evidence it's effective.

Mind-Body Therapies:

- Acupuncture: Studies have shown to be very effective in controlling menopausal symptoms, including sleep.
- Cognitive Behavioral Therapy: CBT and mindfulness have both been shown to reduce menopausal symptoms, including sleep disturbances, hot flashes, and mood instability.
- Hypnosis: While the evidence is inconsistent, hypnosis has been proven effective in controlling symptoms in some studies.

- Yoga: Can be very helpful in pain management, symptom reduction, and improvement in mood and physical resilience.

Keep in mind that supplements and herbs can interact with each other and prescription medications, so always consult your healthcare provider before taking them. Additionally, the benefits of these natural remedies are largely understudied, so proceed with caution.

C Is For Cancer

Sometimes, it does feel like nature somehow has it in for us ladies—first puberty, then menstruation and pregnancy, and then the roaring transition of menopause. But the problems, unfortunately, don't stop there.

Women are also more prone to certain kinds of cancer. While menopause itself doesn't actually increase the risk of developing cancer, as we age, the chances of getting certain types of cancer do go up. Plus, there are some medications used to handle menopausal symptoms that might impact a woman's cancer risk – potentially increasing or decreasing it.

Approximately half of the individuals diagnosed with cancer each year are over the age of 40. If someone in your immediate family (like your mom, sister, or daughter) has or has had breast cancer, especially at an early age, your personal risk also increases. And if you've had a breast biopsy that revealed certain types of benign disease, like atypical hyperplasia, your chances of developing breast cancer are higher, too.

So, what can you do about it?

Well, spotting breast cancer in its early stages, before it spreads beyond the breast, dramatically improves the chances of successful treatment. That's why experts like the American Cancer Society recommend routine screening with a mammogram.

They suggest starting at age 45, but some say waiting until 50 is okay. Your doctor may even recommend starting earlier, depending on your individual risk factors.

Mammograms are designed to catch small abnormalities that can't be seen or felt. But it's important to remember that they don't detect all breast cancers, which is why physical breast exams are also crucial.

The American College of Obstetricians and Gynecologists suggests getting a breast exam every one to three years in your twenties and thirties and then annually once you hit 40.

As for regular breast self-exams, research hasn't shown a clear benefit, but if you choose to do them, make sure to review your technique with a healthcare provider. If you notice any changes in your breasts during self-exams, be sure to report them to your doctor promptly.

If you're at a higher risk for breast cancer, getting a yearly MRI in addition to your mammogram might be beneficial. You could also explore the option of three-dimensional mammography. Taking care of your breast health is important, so stay informed and talk to your doctor about the best screening options for you.

In the end, it is not the female hormones or lifestyle choices that are responsible for the majority of cases of breast cancer. Instead, genetics and family history account for most cases. So, make sure to keep track of your personal and family medical history, and talk to your doctor if you have any concerns.

Now that you're equipped with a deep understanding of hormones and how they impact your menopause journey, let's focus on a topic that bothers many: weight gain. Chapter 3 will guide you through practical and enjoyable ways to manage your weight during menopause. The best part is you won't have to give up the foods you love. Stay tuned for some delicious and healthy tips!

Part II

The Fixes – *Your Menopause Mastery Kit –*
Unchain Yourself from Menopausal Symptoms
With Scientific And Holistic Approaches And
Unleash A Stronger, Leaner, More Vital You

It's time to release the immense power of your new self! With the myths, mis-
conceptions, fears, and limiting beliefs surrounding menopause behind you,
you'll discover a new flow of energy and exuberance. Part II is the core pro-
gram of the book – designed to reboot your body with the latest nutritional
advice and intel on intermittent fasting, exercise routines such as simple yoga
poses, Pilates, strength work, and easy cardio to shed weight, tone up, and
balance hormones. Plus, great sleep hygiene and tips to improve night sweats
and return you to blissful sleep.

Chapter 3

Move, Groove, And Improve

◆◈ ─────────────────────────────────────── ◈◆

IF YOU WERE one of those lucky women who could chow down any food during your early twenties without gaining weight, brace yourself for a harsh reality when you reach your mid-to-late-thirties. During the menopause phase, numerous women encounter an unforeseen opponent: the persistent midlife middle.

As if the hormonal storms and coming to terms with your new reality of menopause and "the transition" weren't enough, our bodies also start to experience some vexing physical changes. And not just small changes here and there. We are talking about a massive overhaul of so many different systems, resulting in a huge shift in our metabolism. In fact, when you actually look at the data, a woman can expect to gain three to five pounds per year during perimenopause and menopause, and no one seems to have a good explanation for that.

For many of us, weight gain may seem unavoidable as we reach middle age. About 85 percent of us will have a sudden, unexplainable increase in weight that has nothing to do with calories in and calories out.

So, is this inevitable?

Are we fighting a losing battle?

Should we just let go of the image of our younger, thinner selves?

The answer is a resounding no! Even though our bodies may be changing, there are still ways that we can take control over how much weight we gain during this transitional period. As Mae West said, *"You are never too old to become younger."*

So, even though you may never have been a fitness enthusiast, it's never too late to start. The key is making lifestyle changes to help manage your hormones and metabolism. For example, getting enough physical activity, making sure you're getting adequate sleep each night, and incorporating stress management techniques like yoga and meditation can help reduce the amount of weight gain related to menopause and improve overall health.

But to understand why so many changes are needed for you to hold on to your health during menopause, it helps to understand what metabolism is and how it works.

Metabolic Mechanics, Menopause And Midlife Middle

Metabolism is the process by which your body converts food into energy to fuel its daily activities. *Cellular* metabolism is the term used to describe all the controlled chemical reactions that take place within a cell.

What is a cell?

For NASA scientists, understanding a cell could be the key to the origin of life. For a chemist, a cell is an intricate and active chemical system, constantly in motion rather than a static entity.

But for the rest of us, a cell is simply the smallest unit of life – your body is made up of over 10 trillion living cells! All these cells need energy, and they get it in two distinct ways: catabolism and anabolism.

Catabolism breaks down large molecules into smaller molecules and releases energy. Anabolism uses this energy to build new molecules. This process is known as cellular metabolism. When we consume an apple, for instance, our digestive system breaks it down, and the resulting molecules are absorbed into our bloodstream and used as essential components for our cells.

After the energy is absorbed and processed, our cells convert it into a type of molecule called adenosine triphosphate (ATP). ATP is like a mini-battery that stores and transports energy within our cells. This energy powers various cellular activities, such as muscle contraction and brain function. The complexity of cellular metabolism is evident through the intricate network of chemical reactions that occur within cells. So, what causes the sudden change in weight during menopause?

Well, for some women, it's the perfect storm.

As we age, the loss of **estrogen** impacts fatty acid breakdown, which can lead to a decrease in ATP production and an increase in oxidative stress. This can further contribute to health issues such as weight gain, inflammation, and fatigue.

This is due to decreasing estrogen levels and declining **testosterone** levels. While testosterone is often associated with males, it is equally crucial for women, albeit in smaller amounts. Testosterone plays a vital role in preserving muscle mass and ensuring a healthy muscle-to-fat ratio in our bodies, specifically for women.

On average, we lose five percent of muscle mass per decade, so we are also not burning as many calories since our metabolism also tends to slow down with age regardless of menopause, leading to a decrease in overall metabolic rate. This means we are burning fewer total calories. This is why many of us struggle to maintain the same energy and physical activity level as we age, even if our diet and exercise habits remain the same.

This can have noticeable effects on both men and women. Men may start to develop a beer belly in their late twenties or early thirties, while women may experience a more abrupt weight gain and thickening around the waist in their mid-forties.

For women, overall weight might even remain the same but redistribute to different areas of their body, typically thickening around the waist. This is a universal experience for women during this transition, regardless of their initial body size.

So, it's important to recognize that this weight gain involves more than just the number on the scale. There are distinct changes happening in our bodies during this period of weight gain.

Another key driving factor is **hunger**.

Ever wonder why hunger strikes? It all comes down to hormones, but not the kind we've been discussing. We're talking about the ones that impact your satiety levels – how full or hungry you feel. They also influence where and how your body stores and burns fat. When these hormones are imbalanced, it's not just obesity that's a concern. Chronic inflammation, heart disease, stroke, diabetes, and more can all come into play. The interplay between these hormones is intricate and varies from person to person.

These hormones are insulin, leptin, ghrelin, cortisol, neuropeptide Y, glucagon, glycogen, GLP-1 (glucagon-like peptide 1), peptide YY, and estrogen and testosterone.

As we age and go through perimenopause, these hormones can cause weight gain in the abdomen. But here's the thing – if you already have insulin resistance, that weight gain may hit you earlier in life. For those with polycystic ovarian syndrome, which is often linked to insulin resistance, the struggle may start even earlier. It's worth noting that *where* you carry your fat can impact your health differently. You see, subcutaneous fat, which is the fat right beneath your skin, does not have as much of an impact on your health as visceral fat, which surrounds our organs.

This type of fat can actually have medical implications and impact internal mechanisms. It's chemically reactive and releases inflammatory mediators right into the body. Surprisingly, even individuals who have a normal BMI and look "thin" can possess excessive visceral fat and relatively low muscle mass. It's called "skinny fat" and is considered the unhealthiest subset out there.

Many people might be misled into thinking they are thin but have a noticeable belly. These fat deposits are associated with some of the leading causes of death, including metabolic syndrome, diabetes, elevated cholesterol and lipids, and cardiovascular disease.

Insulin is another hormone that plays a crucial role in our body, enabling cells to use sugar for energy. However, factors like diet and exercise habits can affect our insulin response, leading to health issues such as insulin resistance. High levels of this hormone can contribute to fat storage and inflammation, especially with a diet rich in sugar and refined carbohydrates.

A study was conducted on young, lean individuals who were in good health. They ate two daily meals consisting of fast food and high calories. The findings revealed a 10 percent increase in weight and a 19 percent increase in fat. Notably, most of these subjects developed insulin resistance. This shows how the quality of your nutrition affects your hormones and their impact on your body.

Leptin and *ghrelin* are hormones that impact fat loss and gain. Leptin regulates energy balance and reduces appetite, leading to fat loss. However, many people develop leptin resistance, just like insulin, where the brain fails to receive the "fullness" signal from leptin. It is designed to prevent overeating, but with leptin resistance, it fails to do its job.

You eat more, you gain body fat. Too much fat means proper leptin signaling is disrupted and worsening insulin resistance. The brain thinks you're starving, which makes you want to eat more. You get fatter, you get hungrier, you eat more, you gain more fat, and so on and so forth. This cycle is why losing weight and keeping it off can be challenging.

On the flip side, when it comes to ghrelin levels, they're at their peak right before a meal and then drop about an hour later. Basically, if we decide to go on a diet and starve ourselves, our body gets hungrier! Even after having a meal, overweight individuals still only have a slight decrease in ghrelin levels, so their brains keep receiving that signal to eat.

This can lead to increased hunger and binge eating.

Next on the list is cortisol, our stress hormone. Like other hormones mentioned earlier, cortisol is crucial for our survival. Cortisol stimulates fat and carbohydrate metabolism for quick energy, promotes insulin release, and maintains blood sugar levels. It is part of our fight-or-flight response. It was designed to boost our energy levels when faced with threats like being chased by saber-toothed tigers. Now, in today's world, stressors are all around us. When this happens, the raised cortisol makes us turn to comfort food for relief, and that can lead to increased fat storage.

All of these hormones work together, taking center stage in the menopause weight game. But here's the real question: does it ever end, or are we destined to pack on the pounds during and after menopause?

No, and no. The numbers won't keep climbing indefinitely. Eventually, they stabilize. However, the "catch" is that the most significant weight gain tends to happen during perimenopause and the years immediately following menopause. And this weight gain isn't just a numbers game – it can profoundly impact your physical health and mental well-being.

Joint Health And The Menopause Spectacle

There are few things that can come between a woman and her active lifestyle, but there is one major exception: joints. If you have an underlying joint condition, it can be difficult to distinguish between menopause-related aches and pains and those caused by arthritis. Although experiencing aches and pains doesn't necessarily indicate arthritis, it is crucial to find out when to seek further assistance and advice.

During menopause, women may be more prone to developing osteo-arthritis, particularly in the hands, and possibly rheumatoid arthritis, too. Osteoarthritis is a result of joint wear and tear, while rheumatoid arthritis is an autoimmune disease. In rheumatoid arthritis, the immune system mistakenly attacks the cells lining the joints, causing swelling, stiffness, and pain.

But what has that got to do with menopause?

The one-word answer is estrogen. It affects both the cartilage, the connective tissue in joints, and bone turnover, the natural replacement of bone in the body. This is why it can contribute to inflammation and pain and why HRT is often prescribed to help reduce inflammation and pain associated with menopause.

The joint pain associated with menopause is quite common. According to a recent survey, nearly 40 percent of women aged between 45 and 65 reported experiencing them. And it can show up even during peri-menopause or post-menopause. Anecdotally, it can even act as an early indication of menopause for some women before the onset of any other symptoms.

Exercise is one of the most effective ways to help reduce joint inflammation and pain. A study examined the impact of a 12-week exercise program on postmenopausal women with osteoporosis. One group performed exercises, including resistance training and balance workouts, while the other did not. After 4 and 12 weeks, the exercising group showed significant improvements in strength and balance and reduced fear of falling compared to the non-exercisers.

So, even if you think you might be hurting your already aching joints, exercise may actually be the key to reducing pain and inflammation. Additionally, it can help keep bones strong and prevent future injury.

The Emotional Journey
Through Body Changes

Your changing body is bound to shake down some emotional and psychological responses. It's a phase where women often feel a shift in their relationship with their bodies. During menopause, our bodies undergo various changes, and it's common to feel a bit unsettled about them. The hormonal fluctuations can cause weight change, alterations in skin texture, and changes in body shape. These shifts might make us feel a little disconnected or even critical of our bodies.

So, how do we accept and move on with our new bodies?

Firstly, it's essential to remind ourselves that these changes are entirely natural. Our bodies are adapting to a new phase, and while it might feel challenging, it's also a testament to the resilience and strength within us. Many previous generations of women didn't even make it to this phase of life.

One way to navigate this is through mindfulness. It's about being present and acknowledging our thoughts and feelings without judgment. When negative thoughts about our bodies arise, practicing self-compassion can help. It's like talking to ourselves as we would to a good friend – with kindness and understanding.

Another aspect is celebrating what our bodies can do rather than solely focusing on how they look. Our bodies have carried us through life's adventures, and during menopause, they continue to support us. Engaging in activities that make us feel good – be it dancing, yoga, painting, or even simply walking – can foster a sense of appreciation for our bodies' capabilities.

Connecting with others going through similar experiences can also be incredibly comforting. Sharing stories, concerns, and laughter with friends or support groups can provide validation and support, reminding us that we're not alone in this journey.

Taking care of ourselves is paramount. Nourishing our bodies with healthy food and staying active not only supports our physical health but also positively impacts our mental well-being. Finding relaxation moments, whether through reading, taking baths, or practicing meditation, is crucial for self-care.

Lastly, let's try to shift the focus from the physical changes to the wisdom and experiences our bodies hold. Celebrate the journey our body has taken, the experiences it has carried you through, and the resilience it exhibits during this phase. Start a Gratitude Journal and log three things each day for a month, and you'll see your confidence soar and your wonder and joy at life's small moments return to you. Practicing gratitude is a powerful way to connect to your heart and feel good about where you're at on your path.

But, in the end, nothing spells self-love as much as the ability to take on the challenge of losing the weight that is bringing you down!

How To Lose The Persistent Pooch

The remarkable thing is that when you look around, losing weight is presented as simply a matter of following a recipe. Drink these shakes, eat these protein bars, skip all carbs, drink gallons of water, avoid all sugars, and you'll lose weight, be happy forever, and you'll never feel insecure in your life again, ever, right?

No.

The thing is that the recipe for success in losing weight is actually quite unique to each individual, like a puzzle to solve. What works for one person might not work for another. It's all about finding the right combination of different tools and nutritional methods (I don't like the word "diet" because dieting is a formula for failure and a prescription for misery), plus willpower, patience, and persistence. So, if you want to lose weight, don't just stick to the same nutritional and exercise routine as everyone else. Find the right combination of lifestyle changes that work for you! Trial and error. Just keep going.

Now that you know how one size does not fit all, and there may be other factors contributing to your weight gain, it's time to look at the management strategies that can help minimize its effects.

Debra Atkinson, a fitness director at a club with three locations working about 60 hours a week, thought she was in the best shape of her life. Wanting a wider work impact, she took a risk at 49, leaving the security of her stable paycheck to establish her own online fitness business, Flipping 50.

Cue the panic after resigning, worrying about finances, and the pressure to make the business work. And she barely allowed herself to get away from the computer, transitioning from someone who exercised frequently to just walking her dog for stable exercise.

However, as she edited online videos of herself months later, Debra was surprised to see a stronger, healthier, leaner version despite her previous belief that she was already in the best shape. This wasn't how it should be, right? It went against everything she knew about weight gain and fitness. Somehow, she was doing less but seeing better results.

Determined to understand this transformation, she researched to find out if her experience could be replicated.

This was when she discovered that most exercise recommendations were based on studies on men, with only a tiny percentage focused on females. These studies mainly involved young, athletic males in their peak muscle mass, a far cry from middle-aged women in menopause dealing with increased fat storage.

Through her own experience, she found that doing less was more, at least for her. She realized that the standard way of working out – often and a lot – wasn't necessary for her.

"What I stumbled on accidentally about myself began to ring true as I poured over research and began coaching clients and saw the same kind of results," she said. "It's not at all what you're thinking: it's not all high-intensity exercise. Nope, the results were astounding, and the signs and symptoms of each client pointed to a unique combination for each client. Some only did yoga," she explains.

Debra said it herself, it's all about finding the perfect balance. Everyone is different and has different needs. That's why finding the right balance of exercise, nutrition, and stress management that works for you is crucial.

Regular exercise has been proven to boost metabolism, improve strength and flexibility, and even help with stress management. But it's also important to find an exercise routine that fits into your lifestyle and is something you enjoy doing. It may mean experimenting with different types of exercise or choosing to do less than what everyone else around you are doing.

A study was done to observe the effects of physical activity on leptin. They fed two groups of people the same thing: one group did aerobic exercise while the other group was asked not to exercise.

In the end, they measured their leptin levels. And guess what?

Leptin resistance was less in the people who did regular exercise. So, engaging in physical activity, such as aerobic exercise and strength training, can assist in weight loss and maintaining a healthy body weight. Building muscle improves calorie burning so that you can shed those extra pounds more easily.

Other than weight loss, exercise is also important for its many physical and mental benefits. A recent study found that just 22 minutes of moderate to vigorous physical activity (MVPA) per day can significantly reduce the risk of premature death caused by a sedentary lifestyle. This study tracked nearly 12,000 individuals aged 50 or older across multiple fitness tracker-based studies and discovered that even a short duration of exercise provided notable health benefits.

Among those who exercised for less than 22 minutes daily, sitting for more than 12 hours daily was linked to a 38 percent higher risk of death compared to sitting for 8 hours. While the World Health Organization recommends 150-300 minutes of weekly exercise, this study suggests that 22 minutes a day can have a meaningful impact.

Dr. Edvard H. Sagelv, the study's lead author, stressed that even minimal exercise can significantly reduce the risk of mortality compared to a sedentary lifestyle. However, there are still health benefits associated with exercise beyond 22 minutes, with no apparent upper limit.

Although the study focused on older individuals, experts point out the wide-ranging benefits of physical activity on mental health, cardiometabolic profiles, cognitive functions, and overall well-being across all age groups. Exercise also promotes better sleep and reduces anxiety and depression.

Researchers emphasized that there doesn't seem to be a limit to the benefits of exercise. However, the risk reduction might level off with longer durations, especially for those with prolonged periods of inactivity. And you know what? Breaking exercise into short bouts throughout the day, also known as "exercise snacking," can be just as beneficial. It makes it easier to fit into your daily routine.

Ultimately, any amount of moderate to vigorous physical activity adds to your overall health, so it's always a good idea to try and squeeze in a bit more activity whenever you can.

Active Aging And Fitness Routines

Doing nothing is easy. But it makes you feel worse in the long run. Instead, a fitness routine can help improve all the problem areas we discussed. Let's look at all the exercises you can do to stay active as you age.

Strength Training

Strength training exercises can be challenging, but Mary experienced their transformative effects firsthand. After her father's passing, her weight reached 290 pounds, limiting her ability to perform daily tasks without becoming breathless. Determined to make a change, Mary joined a gym, where she worked with a personal trainer three times a week.

Initially, Mary faced difficulties performing exercises like jumping with both feet off the ground, crab crawling, bear crawling, full sit-ups, and push-ups due to her weight. However, she persevered and successfully shed over 100 pounds. Inspired by her progress, Mary's friends and family joined the gym, forming a group called the Golden Girls. They now work out together on Sunday mornings and even participate in races to raise funds for local community programs and charities.

Strength training exercises should ideally be performed at least twice a week. They contribute to developing and maintaining muscle mass, boosting strength, and reducing the risk of chronic diseases. Increasing the intensity of your workout routine is often necessary to achieve weight loss or specific fitness goals.

Selene Yeager's *Next Level* book outlined five recommendations for an effective fitness plan, one of which was to lift heavy. She recommended sets of three to five reps of an exercise, repeating that a few times with ample rest. This helps maintain muscle and strength with age, improves bone density, and can lower blood pressure. She suggested hitting a strength-based session where you're lifting heavy two to three times a week at least to see progress.

Switching up your routine can motivate you to keep going and help prevent plateaus. Mixing up a few types of exercises like weightlifting, bodyweight exercises, or HIIT (High-intensity interval training is a protocol alternating short periods of intense or explosive anaerobic exercise with brief recovery periods until the point of exhaustion) can help.

Adding new moves into the mix will also challenge your muscles, which is necessary for growth.

A randomized controlled trial involving postmenopausal women aged 45-70 showed that supervised HIIT exercise training improved bone density and muscle performance. The study suggests potential benefits in managing health concerns like osteoporosis and muscle strength. Another study showed how weight loss with HIIT exercise can improve insulin resistance in obese and overweight individuals.

Aerobic Exercise

Aerobic activities like brisk walking, running, swimming, and cycling can help shed weight and boost energy levels. To achieve this, it is recommended to aim for 30 minutes of exercise five days a week or to spread it out over several shorter periods. Think of it as 150 minutes of walking or 75 minutes of jogging per week.

One recommended approach is sprint interval training, which involves working at a very high intensity for a short period of time, followed by rest and for example, sprinting for 8 seconds and resting for 12 seconds, repeating this cycle multiple times. This can be done in a way that allows for high intensity. Resisted sprinting in the gym can also be beneficial, as it combines hard output with rest and recovery. This can help release hormones that act in place of estrogen, reducing symptoms like weight gain and mood disturbances during menopause.

Another suggestion is to incorporate plyometrics into your routine. Plyometrics involves performing jumping-like activities that put force through your body tissues. These can include jumps, skater jumps, or exercises like third knee highs. Incorporating these exercises in various sessions throughout your week, not just during running, will provide different healthy strains on your body and promote overall strength and agility.

Yoga

Sue, a 60-year-old from Los Angeles, went through menopause and had a bunch of symptoms. It all started with constipation, which messed up her routine as a school teacher. To deal with bloating, she had to get up earlier to go to the restroom and get ready for her classes. Even though she struggled to fall asleep, she had to keep teaching.

The tricky part was her mood swings, and it was only when her kids mentioned it that she realized something was amiss. On top of that, menopause brought weight gain and other bothersome physical changes. This is where yoga helped her. Learning yoga not only kept her active but fulfilled her.

Pretty much anyone can practice yoga. Regular yoga practice can help you improve overall physical health, including increased strength and agility, improved posture, better balance, and more flexibility. It can also reduce stress and anxiety while improving emotional well-being. Plus, it can be a great way to connect with yourself and find peace in moments of distress.

Recent studies have even found that yoga has psychological benefits during menopause. One review looked at four trials with 582 participants and found that yoga improved mood, reduced stress, and enhanced sleep quality and overall well-being. It also showed that yoga and mindful meditation are linked to higher serotonin levels, a neurotransmitter that affects mood and emotions.

Wall Pilates

Pilates is another fantastic exercise choice for women going through perimenopause and menopause. It's gentle but effective, helping to improve flexibility, balance, muscle strength, and endurance. However, if you have any pelvic floor issues or health concerns, it's always a good idea to consult with a physiotherapist or doctor before jumping into intense core movements.

These Pilates mat exercises offer a great starting point if you're interested. All you'll need is an exercise mat to get going.

The Hundred: Focuses on core strength by lying flat on the mat, engaging abdominals, and performing specific arm movements while maintaining abdominal contraction. Variations exist to intensify the challenge for lower abdominals.

Roll Up: A core exercise that enhances spinal mobility and control. It involves lying flat, engaging the abdominals, and gradually peeling the spine off the mat while reaching forward.

Side Kick: Concentrates on hip joint muscles and core strength. It involves lying on one side, lifting and pulsing the leg forward and backward while maintaining a stable spine.

Saw: Increases spinal rotation and strengthens back extensors, promoting upper body flexibility. Requires sitting with legs extended, rotating the upper body, and reaching toward each foot.

Spine Stretch: A stretch that enhances lower back flexibility and spinal mobility while working on abdominal muscles. It involves sitting tall, reaching forward, and articulating the spine sequentially.

These are helpful for premenopausal and menopausal women due to their low-impact nature and multiple benefits, including core strength, flexibility, and spinal health. When done regularly, they can improve posture, increase energy levels, and reduce the physical and mental strain associated with menopause. Additionally, these exercises can also help reduce the frequency of hot flashes.

Having said that, HRT is still the gold standard for managing many menopausal symptoms. A study found that menopausal women using hormone therapy tended to have less body fat, especially the type around the organs (called visceral fat). However, the effect on body fat disappeared once they stopped this therapy.

The research, involving about 1,500 women aged 50 to 80, showed that women currently using hormone therapy had a lower percentage of body fat compared to those who had used it in the past or never used it at all. The study suggests that while hormone therapy might have some impact on body fat while being used, this effect doesn't last once the therapy stops. That is where incorporating a healthy lifestyle, exercise, and diet comes into play.

Who doesn't want to be confident in their own skin again? The best part is that it's never too late to start, even if you've never done it before. You don't have to exercise every single day, but staying active and incorporating weight-bearing exercises and strength training into your routine can work wonders.

I can speak personally here with genuine authority. I was a real couch potato. It's true I had some serious health challenges but getting off my butt and exercising at least three-four times per week (especially when I didn't feel like it) has changed my life! I've lost more than 40 pounds, changed what I eat, and now actually enjoy lifting weights, doing light cardio (on a stationary exercise bike) and going to the gym. It's a lot easier than I imagined.

Menopausal weight gain made me miserable. None of my clothes fit me and I hated my reflection in the mirror. Taking charge of what you eat and how you move changes more than your appearance – you feel mentally more resilient and confident. But don't take my word for it, try it for yourself.

Now that you know the exercises to shed weight, let's move on to the next chapter, which discusses the ideal weight-loss diet plan. The best part? You won't even have to give up your favorite foods. You can still enjoy all the foods you love with intermittent fasting – rather than tedious calorie counting!

Chapter 4

Ditch The Weight, Not The Cake

LET ME INTRODUCE you to Jane. Picture her as a vibrant woman in her mid-40s who always took pride in her active lifestyle. She loved jogging in the crisp morning air, dabbled in yoga on weekends, and relished the culinary arts. For years, her reflection in the mirror had been a trusted and familiar one. However, as Jane transitioned into menopause, something peculiar started happening. Her once-reliable jeans didn't zip up as easily, and each morning, she was greeted by a softer and rounder version of herself.

Frustration mounted as she realized that her trusted exercise routine and healthy eating habits were no longer enough to keep her middle-age "middle" in check.

Menopause had changed the rules of the game.

But she was not alone.

Jane's story mirrored that of countless other women who struggled with menopausal weight gain. (Me included!)

Typically at its worst during the onset of menopause, weight gain can continue to be a problem for the rest of a woman's life.

As Goldie Hawn said, "What helps with aging is serious cognition – thinking and understanding. You have to truly grasp that everybody ages. Everybody dies. There is no turning back the clock. So the question in life becomes: What are you going to do while you're here?"

So, what did Jane do to shift her reality?

Well, instead of just exercising, she adopted intermittent fasting. And whenever she ate, she made sure it was nutrient-dense and healthy.

These two strategies allowed her to manage her menopausal weight gain and maintain her desired shape. If you're like Jane, it's time to get control of your middle-age spread and make the most out of menopause!

Cracking The Code Of Intermittent Fasting

When we are discussing fasting, one thing is sure: we're not talking about starvation! Instead, the goal here is to talk about the specific health benefits of therapeutic fasting.

After extensively reviewing the medical literature, it's obvious that fasting has been used as a therapeutic tool in various cultures and medical systems throughout history. When you look back at the Greeks, Romans, and various cultures worldwide, fasting has been utilized for religious purposes and more for thousands of years.

But here's the thing – we need to be able to tell the difference between evidence-based information and stuff influenced by commercial interests. Fasting is a method that doesn't cost a dime and is accessible to almost everyone. It might not be for everyone, but for those interested in its potential health benefits, it can be a game-changer.

Over the years, we have gained extensive information about fasting and its historical use. Only recently have we begun to comprehend its medical and health benefits truly. Now, let's discuss the physiological aspects of fasting.

Physiologically, when we fast, our body's preferred method of burning fuel is carbohydrates. After consuming a meal with protein, fat, and carbohydrates, *carbohydrates* are burned first for quick energy. Think of them as the first in line to fall.

The process of storing fuel is completely natural and essential for our bodies. It allows us to continue functioning when our carbohydrate reserves are depleted, preventing any adverse outcomes. So, first, we use whatever glucose is floating in our bloodstream. Once we burn through glucose that is readily available from our last meal, our body turns to the liver to release glycogen, the stored form of glucose. And that is then converted into energy for fuel.

Once you burn through the glycogen, the body gets into the "What are we going to do now?" mode. So, it turns to breaking down *fat* into component fatty acids, which are then used for fuel.

It takes about 12 hours for most individuals to deplete the carbohydrates from their last meal. It's important to note that at this 12-hour mark, we begin to experience some of the benefits.

This is the good stuff where we start seeing the health benefits of burning through the bane of our existence: the fat.

So, what are the types of fasting regimens that we can adopt?

The most popular types of intermittent fasting include the 16:8 Method, Alternate Day Fasting, 5:2 Diet, and Eat-Stop-Eat.

The **16:8 Method** involves eating within an 8-hour window each day and fasting for the remaining 16 hours. This method has several benefits, including promoting weight loss, reducing calorie intake, and improving focus and concentration by boosting energy levels during the fasting period. However, it may be too restrictive for individuals accustomed to eating throughout the day.

Another method is the 12 and 12 fasting strategy, which involves eating for 12 hours and fasting for the other 12. This type of fasting is less restrictive than the 16:8 Method, making it a good choice for beginners who are not used to long fasts.

However, it's important to note that this approach may not offer the comprehensive advantages of a 16-hour continuous fasting period.

Numerous studies have consistently focused on a fasting interval of 16 hours, followed by an eight-hour eating window, as the sweet spot for burning fat while preserving muscle.

Additionally, there are quite a few studies that have looked into the benefits of a **5:2 fasting plan**. This plan involves two days of extreme fasting, where you limit your calorie intake to a maximum of 500 calories in a 24-hour period. On these two days, you really have to restrict what you eat. But the other five days, you can eat whatever you want!

This specific fasting pattern has actually shown some really great health benefits. However, many report it's hard to keep up for long periods of time. So, if you're looking to jumpstart your weight loss journey or even improve your overall health and well-being, this could be a great plan for you.

Alternate Day Fasting involves alternating between days of complete fasting and days of eating normally. This method is beneficial in that it can help reduce calorie intake significantly over time, resulting in weight loss. However, it can be difficult to stick to this method if you're not used to fasting for such long periods of time.

Lastly, the **Alternate Day Modified Fasting** method involves consuming 20-25 percent of your normal caloric intake on fasting days and eating normally on non-fasting days. This method is beneficial in that it can provide many of the same benefits as complete fasting without requiring complete abstention from food every other day.

Whichever method you choose, it is important to ensure you get all the necessary nutrients your body needs while fasting. Eating a healthy diet and drinking plenty of water can help ensure that you stay hydrated and nourished while fasting.

One thing to note is that when we talk about fasting, it means *zero calories in a fast*. The misinformation on the internet is when coaches try to sell keto powder and claim, "This won't break your fast."

Let me tell you, after extensive research, I now *know* calories are what break your fast. While your body will utilize whatever you consume as fuel, abstaining from calories means you can have black coffee, tea, and water for hydration – that's it! Chewing gum, and flavored waters, for example, will break your fast. Although black coffee contains minimal calories and a hint of oil from the coffee beans, it will not break your fast. Done correctly, fasting can provide numerous health benefits.

In order to help you manage your menopausal symptoms, fasting needs to be done correctly or not at all. Sound a bit draconian? I promise it's not. If you stop eating around 6 p.m. at night and don't eat again until 8 a.m. or 10 a.m. in the morning, it's not a hardship (well, it hasn't been for me and many others who report its weight loss and maintenance benefits).

Hormonal Harmony Through Intermittent Fasting

Menopause signals the end of a woman's reproductive years. However, as we have seen previously, this doesn't mean your hormones are no longer active. It just means they are performing in a different way. Fortunately, this is where the magic of intermittent fasting comes into play. It can help control the hormone disruption and bring your body back into balance.

It becomes especially relevant when we think about how being over-weight or possibly obese in early adulthood increases your risk of irregular periods and fertility disorders like polycystic ovarian syndrome (PCOS). This happens to be the most common endocrine disorder in women – it's so common, in fact, that you probably know someone in your circle who has PCOS.

A recent study on women with PCOS found that stress neurohormone (like cortisol) levels are consistently elevated in people with this condition. If you're dealing with PCOS, you may be familiar with this. Short-term calorie restriction, such as daily intermittent fasting, has been shown to address some ovulatory consequences in women with PCOS. Therefore, daily intermittent fasting could be a regular part of your protocol if you have PCOS.

This also holds true during perimenopause and menopause as it helps *reduce insulin levels* and *lower fasting glucose levels*, both of which can help you lose weight.

A recent pilot study indicated that periodic fasting diets, like intermittent fasting, simultaneously *decrease the risk factors and biomarkers related to cancer.* The simplest reason is that fasting is associated with decreased inflammation, which has been linked to increased cancer incidence. For those with a high-risk family history of these cancers, adopting daily intermittent fasting into your routine might be beneficial in decreasing your cancer risk. Not to say that you're never going to get cancer, but you can improve your risk factors and increase your chances of survival using a restricted diet.

Aging and menopause also go hand in hand with musculoskeletal conditions like osteoporosis and sarcopenia. These can truly have an overwhelming impact on someone's life. When your bones and muscles don't function properly, it affects your mobility, causing pain and hindering simple activities like lifting grandchildren or moving freely. It's a cycle – if you hurt, you can't sleep, and it cascades into a whole range of psychosocial issues. And the aches and pains of menopause can further compound the problem.

The good news is that fasting has shown promise in *improving bone health* by affecting the secretion of parathyroid hormone. This hormone plays a significant role in calcium and phosphate metabolism. It has also been found to help alleviate symptoms of rheumatoid arthritis by reducing food intolerance, improving gastrointestinal permeability, and reducing the intake of inflammatory mediators like cytokines, prostaglandins, and leukotrienes.

In fact, studies have shown that fasting for seven to ten days can significantly reduce pain, stiffness, and reliance on pain relievers in rheumatoid arthritis patients compared to control groups.

Interestingly, it is also being recognized as a potential strategy to address metabolic abnormalities associated with conditions like metabolic syndrome. These are commonly seen in individuals with apple-shaped bodies, which are characterized by high blood pressure, elevated cholesterol, increased risk for heart disease and stroke, and higher levels of triglycerides.

One prominent effect is the *reduction in belly fat*, which in turn contributes significantly to reducing inflammation. Studies have shown fasting for four weeks can reduce total body weight. A study conducted in 2014 found that following this eating pattern can result in a weight loss of approximately three to eight percent over a period of 3-24 weeks. This is a significant amount when compared to most weight loss studies.

However, what's notable is the impact on body mass index (BMI) and waist circumference. Waist circumference is a critical measure of belly fat and is directly associated with long-term health outcomes. And get this – the same study also revealed that people experienced a decrease of about four to seven percent in their waist circumference. This implies that they lost a *significant* amount of that harmful belly fat that tends to accumulate around our organs and cause various diseases.

Therefore, even if the overall weight loss might not be substantial in a short period, the positive influence on BMI and waist circumference holds considerable importance for long-term health benefits, particularly in terms of reducing abdominal fat.

Fasting has also shown incredible effects on mental health. It can help *reduce symptoms of anxiety and depression*, improve social functioning, and even diminish stress. And the best part? It's completely free! There are several proposed neurological mechanisms that explain how fasting influences mood. It helps neurotransmitters work better, enhances sleep quality, and boosts the synthesis of neurotrophic factors that support brain health.

Clinical observations have shown that fasting can have an early effect on depressive symptoms, leading to improved mood, increased alertness, and a sense of calm. Fasting has also been found to be especially beneficial for reducing brain fog, especially in the mornings.

These are just a few ways fasting can alleviate the various symptoms of menopause. Apart from that, fasting triggers remarkable changes in the body. Hormones like Human Growth Hormone (HGH) skyrocket and boost fat burning and muscle building while increased insulin sensitivity allows for easier access to stored fat. The body also undergoes cellular repair, eliminating old proteins through autophagy. Notably, genes are influenced to promote longevity and protect against diseases. These incredible transformations contribute to the health benefits of intermittent fasting.

Debunking Intermittent Fasting Myths In Menopause

As with anything in life that you can do for free, there are bound to be myths. Intermittent fasting is no different. It's important to take note of the facts so you don't miss out on all the amazing benefits it offers.

Many of the claims regarding fasting during the menopausal transition are often opinions without empirical evidence. And our goal should be not to get dissuaded from considering this extremely beneficial option by marketing tactics.

Myth 1: Fasting Will Make You Gain Weight Faster

It may have already crossed your mind that belly fat and inflammation are linked to "stress," which, as we said, raises cortisol. Therefore, it seems logical that intermittent fasting would also increase cortisol because it puts our body under significant stress, right?

You're right, fasting does lead to a minor increase in cortisol, *but* it's not typically to a level that's considered pathological. We know that the primary factor that raises your cortisol levels isn't fasting; it's stress.

Interestingly, a little bit of stress from fasting is actually a good kind of stress. Our bodies benefit from a certain amount of stress to encourage our biological pathways to become stronger and more resilient.

Cortisol is a crucial survival hormone – our body's fight-or-flight response. Back in the day, it helped us escape from dangers like spear-wielding Neanderthals. Nowadays, those extreme stressors are rare, but our bodies still respond to daily stressors, leading to a chronic, low-grade elevation in cortisol levels.

The issue arises when we're constantly bombarded with stressors from various sources like news, social media, work, and daily life. This chronic stress keeps our cortisol levels consistently elevated, affecting our well-being. However, activities like exercise temporarily raise cortisol levels but actually help lower them in the long run. They act as stress relievers that bring down cortisol levels over time, contributing to better overall health.

Myth 2: Fasting Will Make Menopause Worse

There's another myth going around that intermittent fasting can disrupt women's hormones. But guess what? A review of recent studies from 2022 found that fasting **didn't negatively impact** estrogen, gonadotropins, or prolactin levels in women.

Now, for men, it turns out that intermittent fasting might slightly lower testosterone levels in young, physically active guys, especially if they're on the lean side. But here's the interesting part: this reduction in testosterone doesn't seem to affect muscle mass or strength negatively.

A study led by nutrition professor Krista Varady for the National Institute of Diabetes and Digestive and Kidney Diseases found that women in four-hour and six-hour intermittent fasting groups lost three to four percent of their baseline weight compared with the control groups, which had almost zero weight lost. However, there was a decrease of about 14 percent in a hormone called DHEA, often used in fertility treatments. Despite the decrease, it remained within the normal range.

Additionally, the fasting group showed improvements in insulin resistance and signs of reduced stress in the body.

So, no, your hormones will not be disrupted in a bad way due to intermittent fasting.

Intermittent Fasting Kickstart Kit

Chances are, you've done intermittent fasting without even realizing it. Picture this: you had a late dinner, slept in, and skipped breakfast until lunchtime the next day. This means you have fasted for more than 16 hours already.

Believe it or not, some people naturally eat this way. They simply don't feel hungry in the morning. And you know what they say – simplicity is key. That's why many people find the 16:8 method to be the most sustainable way of intermittent fasting.

You might want to give it a try first! If you breeze through it and feel amazing during the fast, you might want to level up and try more advanced fasting methods.

How about doing a 24-hour fast one to two times a week with the Eat-Stop-Eat approach?

Or maybe restrict your calorie intake to just 500-600 calories one to two days per week with the 5:2 diet?

Alternatively, you can take a more flexible approach. Simply fast whenever it's convenient for you, skip a meal here and there when you're not hungry or don't have time to cook – no need to follow a structured intermittent fasting plan if it doesn't interest you. You can still enjoy some of the benefits. However, without a structured approach, your body might not become accustomed to the fast, so you may not gain as many benefits.

Whichever approach you choose, remember to stay hydrated throughout your fast. Drink plenty of water and avoid calorie-containing drinks
like juices or sodas. You can also enjoy zero-calorie beverages like herbal
teas or black coffee without milk.

The Power Of Nutrition Nuggets

Not many people are big fans of diets because they can be so stressful
and complicated. Over the years, many different diets have gained traction, but they feel like torture for the foodies because most of us are
hungry, tired, and completely miserable on them.

There's no specific diet that's seen to be really good for menopause. But
one of the easiest ones, one of the best ones to follow and to help support your body and your mind during the perimenopause and the menopause, is the Mediterranean diet.

The Mediterranean diet is considered one of the healthiest in the world,
and people in countries surrounding the Mediterranean Sea have followed it for eons. It's a long-term, adaptable diet that can be suitable for
vegetarians, vegans, or those with specific dietary needs. It emphasizes
vegetables, fruits, beans, legumes, nuts, seeds, and healthy oils like fish
oils or olive oil. There's also a moderate amount of dairy, but alternatives
are available for vegetarians and vegans.

Incorporating herbs and spices adds a glorious taste to the food, while
moderate consumption of red wine is also part of the diet. Moderation
is key when it comes to the Mediterranean diet – there is no need to
restrict calorie intake or food groups, but portion sizes must be kept
in check.

The benefits of this diet cannot be understated – some include:

- **Heart Health:** The diet is rich in healthy fats, which is great
  for the heart. Studies have shown that those following a

Mediterranean diet have a lower risk of heart attacks and heart disease.

- **Weight Management:** With its high-quality protein, healthy fats, and abundant vegetables, this diet helps in controlling weight. It stabilizes blood sugar levels, reducing cravings for sugary foods and preventing blood sugar spikes and crashes that can trigger symptoms like hot flashes, palpitations, and headaches.

- **Symptom Relief:** This diet helps alleviate several menopause-related symptoms – especially hot flashes and night sweats.

- **Brain Health:** Healthy oils crucial for cognitive function, memory, and combating brain fog are abundant in this diet. A study looked into how combining moderate-intensity aerobic exercise with the Mediterranean diet could benefit obese postmenopausal women. And no surprises here, the combination intervention not only improved sex hormones, cognitive functions, and functional abilities but also showed potential for addressing sex hormone deficiency and promoting brain health and longevity in postmenopausal ladies.

- **Bone Health:** The diet provides ample calcium and magnesium, essential for bones and muscles, and especially important for postmenopausal women to prevent conditions like osteoporosis.

- **Digestive Wellness:** Herbs and spices in the Mediterranean diet aid digestion and elimination. Bitters, such as fennel and peppermint, stimulate digestion and nutrient absorption. These herbs are often consumed as a first course in meals to aid digestion consistently.

- **Eating Habits:** The Mediterranean diet promotes a sociable and mindful eating experience, focusing on sitting down, eating slowly, and chewing thoroughly. This approach helps prevent indigestion, reflux, and bloating. Additionally, it takes about 20 minutes of eating for the stomach to signal the brain about feeling full, encouraging the habit of eating slowly and mindfully.

So, how can you seamlessly incorporate the Mediterranean diet into your daily routine?

Start by increasing your vegetable intake to include vegetables in every meal. You can have mushrooms, spinach, or tomatoes in your omelet for breakfast. Consider having a salad as a starter for lunch or dinner to boost your vegetable consumption. (My hot tip here is to check out the recipes of Yotam Ottolenghi. He's done numerous books and is a salad master. Whenever I'm stumped for ideas, I thumb the pages of his books for inspiration).

It's also important to be conscious of your fruit consumption, adjusting the quantity based on personal preference and how it affects your blood sugar levels. Some people prefer to have fruit only occasionally, like on weekends, but fruits also serve up a ton of good fiber, boost your anti-oxidant levels and, most importantly, add pleasure to the palate – living long has a lot to do with pleasure, happiness and joy along with satiety. For proof, just look at the Italians, some of the longest-lived people in the world who have mastered the secrets of the Mediterranean diet! They don't stint on things we all love, such as cheese and pasta, but they do eat them in moderation and balance them with legumes and anti-oxidant-rich vegetables.

Another aspect of the Mediterranean diet is to limit red meat to a couple of times a week. Additionally, it's recommended to include oily fish like salmon, mackerel, or sardines in your meals as they are rich in beneficial fish oils and contribute substantially to the Mediterranean-style diet.

Don't forget to add nuts and seeds to your diet, too, as they are high in protein, calcium, magnesium, and healthy fats. You can sprinkle them on salads and soups or include them in your morning porridge. For vegetarians or vegans, incorporating plenty of beans and lentils in stews, soups, and other dishes is highly recommended.

Lastly, cutting out "white" foods such as white bread, rice, and sugar can have a significant positive impact. That said, sourdough bread boosts the microbiome, improves digestion, and has a lower glycemic index than normal white bread. Opting for whole grain or other plant-based alternatives provides more nutrients and benefits. It's also worth mentioning that practicing slow, mindful chewing during meals can greatly contribute to your overall well-being, positively impacting digestion and overall health.

Stress Lowering Snacks

As we discussed in the previous chapter, stress is a significant concern for many of us. Continuous exposure might lead to dangerous levels of cortisol in the blood that end up making you gain weight instead of losing it. But munchies can strike anyone at any time, so it's helpful to have healthy snacks on hand that will help you stay calm and reduce stress levels. Fortunately, there are some delicious snacks that can help eliminate stress and give our bodies and minds a well-deserved break.

- **Dark Chocolate:** Two studies of 95 adults showed that consuming dark chocolate reduced their cortisol levels in response to a stress challenge. Choose dark chocolate with at least 70 percent cacao and watch the amount of added sugar. The downside to this is that it can be high in calories, so you'll need to watch your calorie intake.

- **Black And Green Tea:** A study of 75 men found that drinking black tea decreased cortisol in response to a stressful task compared to a different caffeinated drink. The side effects of tea are minimal but watch out for added sugar if you buy it pre-mixed.

- **Probiotics**: Probiotics are friendly symbiotic bacteria found naturally in yogurt, sauerkraut, kimchi, and more. Some studies suggest that probiotics can reduce cortisol levels when under stress. Some people may experience bloating or gas when taking probiotics, so it's best to start with a smaller dose and work your way up or, better still, get your pre- and pro-biotics from foods such as yogurt, kefir, kimchi, and sauerkraut.

- **Omega-3 Fatty Acids:** Found in salmon, chia seeds, walnuts, and flaxseeds, omega-3 fatty acids have been linked to reduced cortisol levels. Try adding these foods to your diet as part of breakfast or dinner. The side effects are minimal, but watch out for potential allergies.

- **Herbal Supplements:** Many herbal supplements, such as ashwagandha and rhodiola rosea, have been linked to reduced cortisol levels. It's essential to consult with a medical professional before taking any herbal supplements, as they may interact with your other medications.

In moderation, these snacks will not make you lose or gain weight, but they might make you feel better. Especially if you have opted for a rigorous dieting routine, don't forget to set realistic goals and take time out for yourself.

With the right balance of nutrition, self-care, and exercise, you can achieve your health goals in no time! The side-effect is that you'll also look and feel great. You won't believe the anti-aging effects of a few tweaks to your nutrition and exercise regimens. But perhaps the most important part of all these adjustments and changes is that you'll feel a sense of accomplishment and ownership over your life and lifestyle. The word for it is "agency" and when you have it you feel on top of things and as though you've got a grip. Agency equals power and you'll know it when you have it – it's a super-charge to your self-esteem and self-acceptance.

After exploring how intermittent fasting and proper nutrition can help you control weight and harmonize hormones during menopause, it's clear that lifestyle changes are key. These are daytime activities. But what about when the sun sets? In the next chapter, we'll explore how to unwind and enjoy a restful night. You'll find tips for better sleep, relaxation methods, and ways to set the stage for a peaceful evening. Because a good day starts with a good night.

Chapter 5

Into The Tranquil Night

YOU MIGHT HAVE heard the phrase "Sleep is the best meditation" by the Dalai Lama. But if you're like me, you might have wanted to face-palm. The reason: many of us who are on the precipice of the last transition of our lives, or those who are already mid-way into menopause, might find this a lot easier said than done.

Sleep is a particularly tricky business during menopause. Symptoms such as hot flashes and night sweats can leave us feeling exhausted, moody, and anxious, impacting our sleep. For Kathryn, it was much more than just *losing sleep*.

Every woman's journey is different, and the same was true for Kathryn, who lived in the bustling town of Whistler. Her life had seemed blessed running her own gelato company, enjoying skiing adventures, and cherishing motherhood. However, life took an unexpected turn when, in 2016, a cancer diagnosis and subsequent treatments abruptly plunged her into a whirlwind of change. The medication, Tamoxifen, not only targeted the cancer but propelled her into a menopausal spin at an unprecedented speed.

In her own words, "It was like hitting a wall at 100 miles per hour. I shut down." The energetic life she had once led became a distant memory as she grappled with an overwhelming cascade of symptoms, the most debilitating of which, for her, was insomnia.

It robbed her of peace and rest for *years*.

"I would sleep two hours, wake up for two, and repeat," she explained, describing the relentless cycle that seemed to last forever. The lack of sleep wasn't just a single challenge; it brought a flood of mental and emotional struggles.

Her entire identity was shaken. And her story is not unique at all.

On average, about 12 percent of women across all ages face sleep difficulties. But the percentage skyrockets to 40 percent as women progress into their late 40s to early 50s, when they hit – you guessed it – menopause!

That is why this chapter is dedicated to why quality sleep is essential and how effective techniques for better sleep during menopause will save your sanity and well-being. We'll explore lifestyle changes, supplements, and natural methods to improve sleep quality.

The Rhythms For A Restful Slumber

In 1964, Randy Gardner and some college friends, along with University Professor William Dement, decided they wanted to break the world record for the longest period of time without sleep. After just two days, Randy was struggling to keep his eyes open and had difficulty with simple tongue twisters. His friends were also falling asleep against the wall. By day three, he started experiencing coordination issues and mood swings, and by day five, he was hallucinating.

He managed to stay at this zombie level of wakefulness if you can call it that, for 11 days and 25 minutes. And then, he had to be taken to the local naval hospital.

During his first night at the hospital, he slept for 14 hours, with the majority of that time spent in deep and dreaming sleep.

This shows how sleep and mental health are intimately and bidirectionally intertwined. Traditionally, it was believed that sleep symptoms were a symptom of mental health problems. Not the other way around.

However, with more recent studies done on sleep, the understanding is that poor sleep wreaks havoc on neurotransmitters and stress hormones. This, in turn, can cause a variety of mental health problems.

And it is not just mental health either.

Disturbed sleep is further linked to a higher likelihood of cardiovascular events, diabetes, and cancer. Disturbed sleep includes both under-sleepers (those who sleep six hours or less) and over-sleepers (those who sleep ten hours or more), and they both face an "elevated risk of all-cause mortality." Meaning both are more prone to die earlier than if they had been getting adequate sleep.

We're undergoing a healing process when we sleep deep and dream.

So, in this sense, you should consider sleep as your superpower!

However, you have to keep in mind that sleep is not uniform.

On a typical night, most people go through around four to six sleep cycles. Here's the interesting part – not all sleep cycles have the same length, but on average, they last about 90 minutes each.

The first sleep cycle phase is called light sleep, or **Non-Rapid Eye Movement (NREM) Stage 1**. During this stage, your body begins to relax and prepare for entering a deeper sleep state. Breathing and heart rate slow down while muscle tension decreases. You may sometimes experience twitches or jerks as your brain activity transitions to lower frequencies.

You are very easily awakened at this stage.

The second stage of the sleep cycle is **NREM Stage 2**. During this phase, breathing and heart rate slow down and become more regular. Your body temperature drops slightly as your muscles relax even more. You may have brief moments of wakefulness or experience dreamlike images, but most people quickly fall into a deeper sleep.

The third stage is **NREM Stage 3**, also called slow-wave or deep sleep. Brain activity slows down further during this stage, making it harder to wake up. This is when the *glymphatic system*, the brain's waste clearance system, kicks in. It consists of star-like glial cells that synchronize with the cardiovascular system at night. Its job is to remove waste from the brain and provide fresh resources for optimal functioning the next day.

The fourth and final stage of the sleep cycle is **REM (Rapid Eye Movement)** sleep. During REM, your eye movements become more active as your brain processes information from the previous day. This is when vivid dreams or nightmares happen. It also helps clear out unnecessary memories to improve focus on new things.

REM sleep is crucial for learning and memory consolidation.

After REM sleep, the cycle restarts with NREM Stage 1. This cycle typically repeats itself about four to five times throughout the night. Some people may go through fewer or more cycles depending on the length of their sleep.

In theory, since your body was designed to do it, all of this should be simple enough to do, right?

Well, not so much for women in menopause.

We know there are decreases in hormones such as estrogen, progesterone, and primarily testosterone during this phase. These changes are the leading cause of different physiological signs and symptoms that result in sleep disturbances. These show up as vasomotor symptoms like hot flashes and night sweats.

Imagine yourself on a cold winter night when everyone is huddling up in cozy blankets. When you feel like a furnace inside, settling down or staying asleep can be frustrating and difficult.

Other than hormones, our sleep-wake cycle also tends to change and become inconsistent. We start feeling tired earlier and waking up earlier in the morning, resulting in less overall sleep.

But what are these sleep-associated symptoms?

Just as all symptoms of menopause, sleep-associated disorders also vary from woman to woman. Let's look at some of the most common sleeping disorders.

Insomnia

We know for a fact that when someone is drunk, they're definitely not fit to drive. Surprisingly, the same goes for someone who's sleep-deprived. Their performance can be as impaired as if they were drunk. It's something that makes you think about how much importance society places on sleep and how individuals prioritize it.

A study conducted by Williamson and Feyer suggests that going without sleep for approximately 15 to 19 hours can result in behaviors similar to having a blood alcohol level of 0.05, akin to being drunk. Reaction times decrease by 50 percent, and accuracy also tanks significantly.

On average, getting around seven to nine hours of sleep each night as an adult contributes positively to your mood and health, preventing accidents, and even having a successful marriage.

Insomnia is when you have trouble falling or staying asleep on a regular basis – more than three nights a week. People with insomnia often have restless sleep, miss out on overall sleep, wake up early, and feel tired and sleepy during the day. It can make you feel anxious and irritable, and even mess with your focus and memory, and increase headaches and inflammation.

Did you know that one in seven adults deals with chronic insomnia? And for women, that number is even higher – about one in four women experience insomnia symptoms. It gets more common during menopause, with as many as 61 percent of postmenopausal women reporting insomnia symptoms.

I'm literally gagging to tell you that I was one of those 61 percent of postmenopausal women experiencing insomnia. Again, I'm not saying HRT is right for every woman, but it was right for me as it eliminates my insomnia and the palpitations and hot flashes that previously assailed me every night.

Enough about me. Back to the science.

Around 75 to 85 percent of women experience the sizzling sensations of hot flashes during menopause, which can last for a good seven years or even longer.

These mini heat waves can last from a quick 30 seconds to a five-minute roast.

Hot flashes can sometimes turn into night sweats, disrupting your sleep with drenched sheets and body heat. You may experience flushed cheeks and a rush of blood to the face.

Not so pleasant.

Even if you manage to doze off again, the constant awakenings and discomfort result in a serious sleep hangover the next day. In fact, nearly 44 percent of women with severe hot flashes qualify as insomniacs.

Sleep Associated Breathing And Movement Disorders

Another fun little surprise that some may anticipate during menopause is snoring or sleep apnea. *Obstructive sleep apnea* **(OSA)** is a sleep disorder where you temporarily stop breathing during sleep, which can lead to gasping, snoring, and a dip in sleep quality.

Interestingly, research suggests that lower levels of progesterone contribute to the development of sleep apnea because progesterone helps keep the upper airways from relaxing too much, which is what causes those breathing interruptions in OSA.

Other sleep disorders like *restless legs syndrome* and *periodic limb movements disorder* are also linked to menopause. They cause involuntary movements in the legs, which can be uncomfortable, annoying, and disrupt sleep.

So, what does it feel like?

Abnormal sensations like tingling, pins and needles, creeping feelings, numbness, and pain can affect the feet, legs, hands, and arms. Even more disconcerting is that these sensations generally worsen during the evening or when you're in bed. The movements associated with these conditions can also be quite disruptive, causing jerking and kicking of your legs at night.

And these symptoms are actually quite common.

One study, which included 5000 menopausal women, found that around 18.1 percent of women aged 45-54 experienced restless legs syndrome. Interestingly, this percentage increased to 20.9 percent among women aged 55-64.

The cause of these fascinating yet vexing symptoms is largely unknown. One theory is that estrogen levels going up and down can impact levels of dopamine and another chemical called glutamate. Both of these chemicals are neurotransmitters that play a role in how your body moves and feels.

Another theory is that genetics may also play a part, as research has found some links between restless legs syndrome and certain genes. Lastly, lifestyle factors such as smoking and lack of sleep can contribute to restless legs syndrome symptoms.

Mood And Sleep

Menopausal sleep complaints, including difficulties falling asleep or staying asleep, are frequently accompanied by feelings of depression and anxiety. And while it may just be because you can no longer get a good night's rest, researchers have also found that changes in hormones can worsen depressive symptoms.

Let me explain.

Estrogen is involved in metabolizing serotonin and other neurotransmitters that influence our sleep-wake cycle. Plus, it helps keep our body temperature low at night, associated with better sleep. So, when there's less estrogen, we experience higher body temperatures, lower-quality sleep, and a not-so-happy mood.

These emotional factors can further exacerbate the sleep issues experienced during menopause. Hence, addressing both sleep problems and emotional well-being becomes crucial for women going through menopause.

But is this the end, or can you still catch up on sleep?

Actually, yes! Let's look at some of the ways to improve your sleep if you're going through menopause.

Sleep Solutions For Menopausal Women

Cognitive Behavioral Therapy For Insomnia

In the past year, the American College of Physicians (ACP) endorsed CBTI as the first-line treatment, supporting its effectiveness. Fortunately, we have over 30 years of efficacy data showing that cognitive behavioral therapy for insomnia (CBTI) truly works. It is effective not only for menopausal women but also for women with cancer and chronic pain. This behavioral approach has been shown to improve the sleep of approximately 80 percent of individuals.

And it worked wonders for Michelle, too.

46-year-old Michelle Foley was a single mom who worked full-time for a multinational computer company. She juggled a full plate on a daily basis, but her biggest hurdle was she couldn't sleep.

Michelle was averaging about two hours a night and sometimes it was zero. Her struggles with insomnia began in 2012 when her mother became sick. Like many women, she didn't immediately recognize it as insomnia. She thought her fatigue was due to a demanding job and caring for her ailing mother.

Over time, her lack of sleep took a toll on other aspects of her life, affecting her appearance, work, and daily tasks. The impact on her health became evident as she gained 40 pounds, experienced memory lapses during presentations, and found it challenging to perform routine activities, even driving.

Despite her usual independence, she felt anxious and agoraphobic, fearing to stray more than a few blocks from home due to the constant struggle to stay awake.

Michelle's primary care physician referred her to a pulmonologist to investigate sleep apnea. But when she called to schedule, the provider asked if she snored. Unsure of the cause of her lack of sleep, they refused to book an appointment. Frustrated, Michelle checked the primary provider directory, calling everyone associated with sleep. The earliest appointment was in three months. Determined to get help sooner, Michelle pivoted and reached out to a cognitive behavioral therapist for insomnia.

So, what is cognitive behavioral therapy for insomnia and should you pin all your hopes on it?

Cognitive behavioral therapy for insomnia (CBTI) is a form of psychotherapy that focuses on changing unhealthy thought patterns and behaviors associated with sleeplessness. It's based on the concept that your thoughts, feelings, physical sensations, and behaviors are all interconnected. This approach teaches you to manage your responses to stressors to improve your sleep and overall quality of life.

With the help of cognitive behavioral therapy, Michelle was able to identify and address underlying issues that were causing her insomnia, such as stress, anxiety, and negative thought patterns. After just a few weeks of working with her therapist, she noticed a marked improvement in her sleep quality and overall well-being. Her energy levels also increased significantly. Ultimately, Michelle was able to get her insomnia under control and finally get some restorative sleep.

It is important to note that this type of treatment is not a one-size-fits-all solution, and everyone may respond differently or not at all. Research suggests that this form of treatment can be particularly effective for those who suffer from *chronic* insomnia.

In one study in 2016, it was found that 65 percent of women who took the therapy had no symptoms of insomnia after eight weeks. After 24 weeks, that number had risen, indicating a sustained and significant success rate in addressing insomnia symptoms.

In another study conducted in 2018, researchers wanted to find out how cognitive behavioral therapy for insomnia (CBTI) compares to other treatments. They gathered a group of 117 postmenopausal women and split them into different treatment conditions. What they found was that CBTI led to significant reductions in depressive symptoms, especially after six months of treatment. This study highlights the strong link between better sleep and reduced depression.

These results are encouraging and show how effective cognitive behavioral therapy can be for those with chronic insomnia. Working closely with your healthcare provider to create a personalized treatment plan that works best for you is recommended.

And if you can't access CBTI, thankfully, there are other measures you can take to improve your sleep.

Sanctuary Of Sleep

The basic idea of sleep hygiene – optimizing your environment and habits for better sleep – applies to almost everyone. However, the perfect sleep routine can differ for each person.

That's why it's important to experiment with different adjustments to discover what benefits your sleep the most. You don't have to make all the changes at once; even small steps can significantly improve your sleep hygiene.

So, how can you practice good sleep hygiene?

Well, it's all about setting yourself up for a great night's sleep every single night. You need to nail your sleep schedule, your pre-bed routine, and daily habits so that quality sleep becomes second nature. You also need a cozy bedroom environment that lets you relax and drift off.

The upcoming tips aren't strict rules – feel free to adapt them to your own situation.

Set Your Sleep Schedule

Having a consistent schedule is key to making sleep a regular and important part of your day. It helps train your brain and body to get the right amount of sleep. Here are some tips to establish a consistent sleep pattern:

First, try to wake up at the same time every day, even on weekends. This sets a rhythm for your body. Also, make sleep a priority. With so many things vying for your time, it's crucial to prioritize sleep. Calculate a target bedtime based on your wake-up time and aim to wind down around that time each night.

When changing your sleep schedule, take it step by step. Avoid sudden shifts that can disrupt your routine. Instead, make small adjustments of up to an hour or two at a time. This way, you can adapt and settle into the new schedule.

Lastly, be mindful of naps. While they can boost daytime energy, long naps can interfere with nighttime sleep. Keep naps relatively short and limit them to the early afternoon. The Sleep Foundation recommends that the ideal nap time is 20 minutes and no longer than 30 minutes to ensure you don't fall into deep sleep, thereby risking valuable nighttime sleep.

Remember, getting a good night's sleep is vital for your overall health and well-being.

Follow A Nightly Routine

First things first, maintaining a consistent routine is vital. Follow the same steps each night – put on your PJs, brush your teeth, and your mind will know it's time to sleep. Set aside about 30 minutes to wind down. Engage in relaxing activities like listening to soft music, light stretching, reading, or practicing relaxation exercises.

Dim the lights as bright lights can disrupt melatonin production, the hormone that promotes sleep. Create a soothing atmosphere with dim lighting.

Now, an important one – disconnect from electronic devices. Give yourself 30 to 60 minutes without screens before bed. These devices can stimulate your mind, and the blue light they emit can disrupt melatonin production.

Consider exploring different relaxation techniques. Shift your attention to relaxation instead of solely focusing on falling asleep. Meditation, mindfulness, paced breathing, and other techniques can help you prepare for bedtime.

If you find yourself tossing and turning, get out of bed. You'll want to associate being in bed with being asleep. After 20 minutes of restlessness, engage in calming activities in dim light, like stretching or reading, then give falling asleep another shot.

Lastly, your sleep environment also plays a big role when it comes to getting a good night's sleep. Creating a peaceful sleep environment is key for a good night's rest. Factors like a comfortable mattress, cozy bedding, optimal temperature, light-blocking curtains, noise-cancelling options, and calming scents like lavender and chamomile essential oils sprinkled on your pillow can also enhance your sleep experience.

By incorporating some of these tips into your pre-sleep routine, you can relax and make it easier to fall asleep when you want to.

Cultivate Healthy Daily Habits

Other tips include changing your daily habits so you can get better sleep. These include:

Get some daylight exposure to regulate your circadian rhythms.

Stay physically active for better sleep and overall health.

Quit smoking to avoid sleep problems caused by nicotine.

Limit alcohol consumption as it can disrupt your sleep.

Cut back on caffeine in the afternoon and evening.

Reserve your bed for sleep (and other fun activities).

Some of these strategies, like cutting back alcohol, which many people use to help them get to sleep, are easier said than done, but by implementing these techniques, you can really improve your sleep quality and overall well-being. It's not just about bedtime habits; establishing positive routines throughout the day can really help regulate your body's natural sleep-wake cycle and minimize any disruptions.

Nutritional Nudges To Better Sleep

Snooze Supplements

Did your mother ever tell you to drink warm milk at bedtime to help with sleep? Well, it's not just an old wives' tale. Some foods are proven to help promote your body's natural production of melatonin.

Melatonin is a fascinating hormone primarily involved in regulating our sleep-wake cycles, with additional benefits such as anti-inflammatory effects, antioxidant properties, and even anti-aging effects on the skin and eyes.

During menopause, lower melatonin levels can disrupt sleep quality and onset. Supplementing with melatonin shows promise in addressing these concerns, improving sleep and alleviating symptoms of depression and mood changes associated with menopause-induced sleep disturbances.

Melatonin supplementation offers more than just sleep enhancement. It also eases pain related to conditions like arthritis or fibromyalgia, enhances bone density (which can be impacted during menopause), and supports healthy body mass.

B vitamins are also extremely important when it comes to supporting sleep during menopause. These vitamins help with energy production, forming red blood cells and ensuring the heart and nervous system work properly. If you're lacking in certain B vitamins, it can make menopause symptoms like hot flashes and mood swings worse. Take vitamin B6, for example. Getting enough of it through your diet or supplements might actually help ease the severity of hot flashes. Folic acid in specific doses has shown promise in reducing how intense and how often those hot flashes happen.

Another supplement that has gained traction in recent years is **magnesium**. It is involved in many bodily functions and plays a crucial role in regulating sleep. Research suggests that getting enough magnesium may improve sleep quality and help with symptoms like mood changes and depression during menopause. It is also important for maintaining bone health, which is especially relevant during menopause. In fact, a 2021 study showed a significant increase in hip, femoral and neck bone density in 80 percent of participants on 500 mg of magnesium – potentially very good news for 8.9 million people who have an osteoporotic bone fracture worldwide each year.

Another study conducted by Alateeq et al. in 2023 looked at how dietary magnesium intake relates to brain health in middle-aged to early older adults. And guess what? The findings showed that people who consumed more magnesium had bigger brain volumes, regardless of gender. But here's the interesting part – the neuroprotective effect of magnesium was particularly noticeable in post-menopausal women. So, overall, it seems like having a higher dietary magnesium intake can be pretty good for brain health, especially for women.

Beyond these commonly discussed supplements, options like *black cohosh* and *valerian root* have garnered attention for managing menopause symptoms, particularly hot flashes and night sweats. However, evidence supporting their efficacy remains inconclusive, revealing the need for further research.

While these supplements hold promise, caution is crucial. The lack of regulatory oversight for supplements implies potential risks and interactions with medications.

But where do you go if you don't want to opt for the supplements?

To the source, of course.

Slumber Snacks

Some excellent options to consider include nutrient-rich spinach, leafy greens, avocado, cashews, dark chocolate, almonds, pumpkin seeds, bananas, and protein-packed beans. These foods are also rich in vitamins, minerals, and essential compounds like phytoestrogens.

Certain foods can naturally help our bodies produce melatonin. Two specific foods known for promoting melatonin are milk and tart cherry juice. A recent study found that these foods benefit all age groups, improving sleep onset, quality, efficiency, and duration.

Milk contains high levels of tryptophan, an amino acid that contributes to melatonin production. In Ayurveda, the ancient Indian system of medicine, warm milk has been used for centuries to promote healthy sleep. Instead of thinking of this as a medicine or supplement, try enjoying this sleep-promoting beverage. Warm up the milk on the stove and consider adding cinnamon, cardamom, or turmeric for flavor. Drink it about an hour or two before bedtime to enhance sleep and address nighttime munchies. If you can't consume dairy or choose not to, oat milk is an excellent alternative that is high in tryptophan and melatonin.

Another food mentioned for promoting sleep is tart cherries. These cherries are rich in tryptophan and melatonin and have been traditionally used to aid sleep. A trial found that participants with insomnia who drank 16 ounces of tart cherry juice daily for two weeks slept an average of 85 minutes longer.

The next is kiwi fruit, which is considered a superfood. Kiwis contain high levels of serotonin, a neurotransmitter involved in various bodily functions, including sleep. A study from Taiwan revealed that participants who ate two kiwi fruits an hour before bed every night for four weeks experienced improved sleep parameters.

Walnuts, also a superfood, are rich in docosahexaenoic acid DHA, an omega-3 fatty acid beneficial for the brain. They also contain fiber, vitamin E, magnesium, prebiotics, and antioxidants. Walnuts are easily absorbed and are a great source of melatonin. Including walnuts in a well-balanced diet can contribute to brain health, mood regulation, and reduced rates of depression.

Digestion And Sleep

There's a whole range of foods and drinks that can disrupt your sleep, and there are also foods that can help improve your sleep. However, it's not just about the food itself; digestion plays a crucial role. During perimenopause and menopause, changes in estrogen levels can affect digestion, slowing it down and making it more challenging to process food. This slowdown in digestion, especially of heavy meals, consumes significant energy, making them less ideal, particularly at night.

We're going to focus on foods that aid digestion during the night, preventing disruptive churning. These foods support digestion and have a calming effect on the nervous system, and may even trigger sleep-inducing hormones. This approach aims to reduce stress on the digestive system and provide healing, calming foods for better sleep. Opting for lighter evening meals is advisable, but if hunger strikes later on, night-time snacks can be crucial during menopause.

Contrary to conventional advice, stabilizing blood sugar levels is paramount, as low blood sugar in the middle of the night can contribute to sleep disturbances. Maintaining stable blood sugar during the night can positively impact sleep.

Let's focus on healthy snacks; most are around 100 calories, making them weight-friendly. These snacks won't adversely impact your weight. The recommended snacks contain protein, healthy fats, and fiber, supporting better sleep. Timing is crucial—consume snacks about an hour and a half to an hour before bedtime to allow ample time for digestion without stressing your system during sleep preparation.

Consider these healthy and low-calorie snacks about an hour and a half to an hour before bedtime:

- **Full-fat Greek Yogurt**: Full-fat Greek yogurt with organic cocoa powder. Top with organic cocoa powder, a handful of nuts and seeds, or some berries.

- **Oat Crackers:** Pair with ordinary cheese, nut butter (such as almond butter or peanut butter), or a nut butter spread without added sugar.
- **Small Sandwich:** Use nitrate-free cold meat, like chicken breast or tuna, a bit of lettuce, and whole-grain bread for a source of fiber, protein, and healthy fats.
- **Sliced Apple:** Spread with nut butter or peanut butter for a delicious combination of fiber, protein, and healthy fats.
- **Avocado:** Half a small avocado with a teaspoon of mayonnaise or cream cheese for a lighter and fresh option.

These snacks provide a variety of nutrients and can contribute to a stable blood sugar level during the night, promoting better sleep. The combination of fiber, protein, and healthy fats will help to keep you satiated until morning.

Cutting Edge And Novel Treatments

During my research for this book, I discovered a few cutting-edge and novel treatments that can help people achieve better sleep. One of these is something called *Fezolinetant*, an oral medication for treating moderate to severe hot flashes in menopausal women. This drug is the first of its kind to receive FDA approval for managing these vasomotor symptoms. It binds to the NK3 receptor, which affects body temperature regulation without relying on hormones. This makes it a suitable option for women who can't use hormone treatments for medical reasons.

The approval comes from the SKYLIGHT 2 trial, which showed that Fezolinetant significantly reduces moderate to severe hot flashes compared to a placebo. The drug's safety warning includes precautions like baseline liver tests and periodic monitoring during treatment. This approval is a big step towards providing non-hormonal treatment options for menopausal hot flashes.

Another step towards the right direction is the use of artificial intelligence. A machine learning algorithm has been developed to predict and alleviate hot flashes in menopausal women using a wearable device called Embr Wave. The algorithm monitors physiological signals to detect early indicators of hot flashes, triggering the device to provide cooling sensations and prevent their onset. While this technology shows promise, further clinical trials are needed to evaluate its safety and effectiveness.

This non-hormonal approach aims to offer an alternative for managing hot flashes, a common symptom among menopausal women who cannot or choose not to undergo hormone therapy.

Fortunately, the field of medicine is ever-evolving, and the therapeutic options are growing. For now, you have the tools to improve your sleep and understand its link to overall health; you're ready to tackle the emotional aspects of menopause. The next chapter will guide you through managing mood swings effectively. Stay tuned to take charge of your emotional well-being.

Part III

The New You – *Reclaim Your Power, Radiate,*
and Rise – *Ignite Your Spirit, Reveal Your True*
Self, and Embrace The Future With A Deepening
Sense Of Self-Love And Self-Compassion

❖◈ ────────────────────────────────── ◈❖

Rediscover your youthful vigor, sexuality and confidence to create a compel-
ling second act in life where you're the unapologetic heroine of your own story.
This part of the book is about reclaiming and expressing your essence, celebrat-
ing your burgeoning self-acceptance and finding the balance you've always
dreamed of. You'll learn how to deal with mood swings, reconnect to your sexy
self, and get insider information on how to make the most of your glorious
assets – your skin, hair, style, and figure to reflect your inner radiance.

Chapter 6

Mood Swings In The Rear View Mirror

AS A WOMAN, you may be familiar with emotions like frustration, gloom, anger, sadness, and anxiety. These feelings are often experienced during PMS. However, when the switch flips unexpectedly, and you notice a disproportionate reaction to something as simple as your partner breathing wrong, you should start questioning if something deeper might be going on.

According to the American College of Obstetrics and Gynecology, 40 percent of women experience mood symptoms during menopause, and it closely resembles the symptoms of PMS. These symptoms may include irritability, low energy, tearfulness, moodiness, or difficulty concentrating.

Unlike PMS, which came before your period, these mood changes come as a surprise.

Let me get this straight. Many women know that pregnancy and periods both come with mood changes that can sometimes escalate to depressive symptoms. However, many women are caught off guard or often overlook the fact that menopause can also cause mood changes.

I know what you are thinking!

Wasn't the whole point of menopause the end of menstruation? And shouldn't you be rid of these mood swings now that the monthly monster is put to rest?

In an ideal world, that should have been the case. But we don't live in that world.

The fact of the matter is that there are many complex hormones at play, and they can still cause havoc even when our periods have stopped. And there can be more triggers that may set off any mood symptom.

So, if you want to throw the nearest object at your partner for breathing too loud, then don't fret. It is quite possible that it is just a sign of the hormonal changes you are going through.

Emotional Ebb And Flow

Each of us is on our unique journey when it comes to the big "transition." And it was just so for Katie. Her journey into menopause began with the surgical removal of her ovaries due to severe endometriosis. Katie had already battled the pain of endometriosis for years, but she hoped the removal of her ovaries and a lot of endometrial tissue would signal the end of her woes. How wrong could she be?

Katie had resented the burdens of being a woman since she was a teenager.

But at 32, she went into early menopause and got every symptom in the book – dry vagina, night sweats, brain fog, sore breasts, reduced sex drive, itches, aches and pains, weight gain – you name it, she got it.

It was not easy.

The worst of it was that she felt incredibly blue and moody, and when she looked in the mirror, she hardly recognized herself. "I saw this much older woman staring back at me. I felt disoriented, depressed and confused. It was truly the worst time in my life."

Peter Scazzero, in his book *Emotionally Healthy Spirituality*, talks about the need to become aware of what is going on around us and *within* us.

In his own words, "Emotions are the language of the soul." But what happens when your body physiologically opposes who you are at your core? You no longer have control over your emotions, and you want to know why this is happening to you.

So, what causes this zero-to-one-hundred reaction?

There's a gland called the amygdala in our brain. It stores our perceptions and feelings of anger, fear, and sadness. It also helps us control aggression and stores memories of past events and emotions, which prepares us to respond if we encounter a similar dangerous or awful situation again.

The problem here is that as our estrogen falls, the *control* of this gland decreases. It's like Pandora's Box. Suddenly, it opens, and you react more strongly and quickly to situations that would normally trigger fear, anger, sadness, or aggression – but at levels you can control.

Another factor is the serotonin in our brain. Serotonin is a chemical that keeps our mood up, makes us happy, and regulates our emotions, but when estrogen levels drop, this hormone can also decrease. As a result, we may struggle to control our emotions and experience rapid mood swings.

It's like this: the less serotonin we have, the less happy we are.

You might find yourself getting easily irritated.
Your patience may decrease significantly.
You might not be able to tolerate certain people anymore.
You may not want to be in the same room or space as people you used to be quite content with.

Sometimes, past emotions can also resurface when triggered. For example, if someone hurt you with their words in the past, that memory is stored in the amygdala. So, when someone says similar words today, even if they don't mean them the same way, your brain recalls that initial instance of anger or hurt. As a result, you may respond based on the past rather than being in the present.

Other triggers can also contribute to mood swings. Stress is a known factor, and let's face it, who isn't stressed these days? Lack of sleep can exacerbate these emotions. Dehydration and low blood sugar levels can also play a role. If you consistently experience the same emotions at the same time each day, it might be an indication that it could be due to dehydration or low blood sugar levels.

The good thing is that "the rage" is usually a phase. It's possibly the imbalance between your hormones and your serotonin levels. But, as your body learns to adjust, you should find that this phase trails off and disappears. And it can also get better if we address all the other contributing factors mentioned above.

Feeling The Blues

Along with rage, there can be lows in the form of depression, which can sometimes be severe. People experiencing depression during this time may find it challenging to control a rollercoaster of emotions. Low serotonin levels play a significant role in this. However, it's important to remember that you're not alone – many women going through menopause feel the same way, and there is help available.

According to a study led by Timur and Sahin, around 41.8 percent of women in the perimenopausal and postmenopausal stages experienced symptoms of depression (that's a lot of women!). Among all women, 23.2 percent were still premenopausal, while 56.9 percent were already postmenopausal. The study also revealed alarmingly that 8.4 percent of women reported having suicidal thoughts.

Menopause specialist and the founder of the website Menopause Matters, Dr Heather Currie, says, "All women experience menopause, with varying severity and duration of symptoms. The described severity [suicidal thoughts and actions], while hopefully uncommon, is sadly not rare. Many women have had their home, social, and work-life devastated by menopausal symptoms."

If you have depressive symptoms or, worse, suicidal thoughts, do not dilly-dally. Go straight to your doctor or the nearest hospital and seek prompt and thorough treatment.

On Pins And Needles

Butterflies in your stomach before a presentation often indicate the importance of the occasion and can be deemed a good stressor. The anxiety associated with menopause is different to the short-term feeling of a churning tummy. Menopause can trigger heightened anxiety beyond every day worries. If these butterflies take over your life and you constantly feel a looming sense of dread, it could be a sign of anxiety. According to Dr. Currie, hormonal changes during menopause can make women more prone to high levels of anxiety.

And there can be different types of anxiety associated with menopause. Some women become more socially anxious, worrying about social interactions or being judged by others. Others worry excessively about health issues, financial obligations, or work-related problems.

The Hidden Emotional Ride Of Menopause

We have discussed the commonly experienced emotional symptoms like rage, anxiety, and the blues. However, there are also lesser-known symptoms that women may not realize are linked to menopause and can cause significant distress. Let's look at those symptoms.

Intrusive Thoughts: This involves a lot of situations that can be challenging to pinpoint. It includes unwanted thoughts randomly popping into your head, impulsive urges that may seem out of character, mental images that trigger anxiety and stress, fears of behaving inappropriately or embarrassingly, concerns about illnesses, and even flashbacks from distant past experiences you'd prefer not to revisit. Additionally, it may manifest as obsessive behaviors, resembling obsessive-compulsive tendencies.

Foggy Memory: Another symptom of menopause is a foggy memory. Incredibly, 60 percent of women report comprehension and memory difficulties after their menopause. This includes difficulty recalling words, focusing on tasks, and remembering simple instructions or information that was once easy to access. While this may be attributed to normal aging, research suggests it can also be linked to decreased estrogen production and menopause. This can result in the doom thinking that you are no longer suitable for your job, your husband no longer loves you, your friends find you irritating, and so on... which leads us to our next symptom.

Heightened Fears: Women can experience intense fear for their loved ones and worry about various situations. Worst-case scenarios dominate their thoughts, making it difficult to see any positive outcomes. It can be related to family, friends, or the world, including current events. If you already have phobias, they can also become heightened, such as fear of spiders, new places, flying, or failure. New fears may arise, like driving in traffic or meeting new people. The desire to go out, socialize, or try new things evaporates. Even familiar activities like travelling may seem daunting.

Loss Of Humor: This is quite a strange one. At some point, we may get tired of people who constantly joke around. We may find their humor is no longer funny, and their personality and sarcasm can irritate us. We might become more sensitive to others' comments, misinterpreting their intentions. As a result, we may lose interest in socializing and prefer to be alone. For example, you'd go out with a group of people and have a great night. But at some point, you sit there, thinking, "Why am I here? These people are annoying me. I don't find any of this fun. I want to go home and be on my own."

Let's be real – all of these symptoms are difficult to pinpoint, but try to remain aware of the changes in our behavior, especially if our loved ones mention it, because we can't always tell if we're having a bad day or something deeper is happening.

How To Keep Calm When You See Red

How many times have you been told:

You're acting crazy!
You need to get a grip!
It's time to calm down!

And how many times has it actually worked? Not often. People telling you to "get a grip" does not actually help you. In fact, it can be downright counter-productive. But once the red haze clears and you realize what you have done or said – you cannot believe it was you. The embarrassment and everything else that goes with it can obviously cause a lot of emotional distress, both to you and to those around you.

So, how do you keep calm when it feels like everything around you is getting out of control?

In the UK, NICE recommends Hormone Replacement Therapy (HRT) as a solution for managing mood swings during menopause. Research indicates that HRT can effectively alleviate symptoms. A 2018 study conducted by US researchers found that women who underwent HRT for a year had a reduced likelihood of experiencing depression during this transitional phase.

But other than HRT, you can adopt various other helpful strategies to keep your emotions in check.

Here are five tips to help you stay calm and balanced during menopause:

Regular Exercise

Our bodies release "feel-good" hormones like serotonin and endorphins when we exercise, which helps us manage stress levels better. Exercising also helps stimulate brain activity and boost concentration.

It can be a great way to release pent-up energy and improve your mood. Activities like boxing, contact sports, or even playing tennis against a wall can help you let off steam. Joining a dance or exercise class provides an opportunity for social interaction and helps maintain bone health during menopause.

In fact, research shows that physical activity can have positive effects on mental health, sometimes comparable to antidepressants. While exercise shouldn't replace antidepressant treatment (if it's warranted), it can boost brain chemicals and improve overall well-being.

Mindfulness And Meditation

Anna was one of the women stressed from the symptoms of her menopause and had to take a few days off work. She was almost on the brink of quitting due to persistent brain fog. She said, "I feel like I'm living in a fog. I just can't think clearly, and it made me feel so overwhelmed with my job and life. It was really affecting my work performance. I knew something had to change."

She discovered profound relief when she began attending relaxation classes, where she learned effective stress management techniques. Surprisingly, hypnosis also played a significant role in her healing journey. She was astounded by the swift clarity of her mind and the newfound sense of control she gained over her life.

Relaxation exercises help relieve stress by promoting a state of calm and easing tension in the body. By practicing deep breathing exercises, you can lower stress levels, increase oxygen intake, and promote relaxation.

Some women have discovered a powerful "paced respiration" technique that can help manage mood symptoms. Paced respiration involves slow, deep breathing, aiming for a gentle rhythm of six to eight breaths per minute instead of the usual 15.

Take a deliberate, slow inhalation while counting to five, then a soothing five-second exhalation. Remember to count purposefully and take deep breaths. Once you become familiar with the technique through a 15-minute session, try incorporating it into your daily routine for 10-15 minutes (some recommend both morning and evening sessions). Whenever you feel out of balance, start your paced respiration and maintain it for five minutes.

Meditation helps you focus and quiet your mind, promoting mental clarity and reducing anxiety. So, if you feel overwhelmed or anxious, try meditation and breathing for a few moments. It can be immensely helpful for managing stress, calming your mind, and improving mental clarity. With regular practice, you can use the skill of mindful meditation to maintain balance in life.

Mindfulness training helps you be present without dwelling on the past or worrying about the future. It creates a space where you're encouraged not to focus on past negative events or fret about what might happen in the future. It also allows you to be grateful for all the good you have right now and reinforces positive feelings.

A recent study explored whether an eight-week program called Mindfulness-Based Stress Reduction (MBSR), which includes meditation and yoga, could help reduce depressive symptoms in women going through menopause. They divided 104 women into two groups: one group received MBSR, while the other group was on a waitlist. Over a period of six months, the study tracked various factors like depressive symptoms, stress levels, anxiety, resilience, and sleep quality.

The results showed that participants in the MBSR group reported fewer depressive symptoms, less stress and anxiety, better resilience, and improved sleep compared to the waitlist group. Interestingly, MBSR had a stronger positive effect on those with a history of major depression or recent stressful events.

You can also use affirmations to help reduce depressive symptoms and improve overall well-being. Affirmations are powerful statements that you repeat to yourself daily in order to change thought patterns and behaviors positively. They can be used as part of a mindfulness practice or on their own. Try saying some of these affirmations out loud in the morning and evening:

- I love myself just the way I am.
- I accept who I am and how I feel today.
- I forgive myself for not being perfect.
- I am worthy of taking up space and being seen.
- I have the strength to get through anything that life throws my way.
- Everything will work out in its own time.

By repeating these affirmations each day, you'll start to believe them, and they'll become part of your reality. When dealing with mood swings and emotional outbursts, the most powerful tool you have is your own mind – use affirmations to help give yourself a positive outlook.

Empathy And Expression

Having a strong support system during menopause is incredibly important. It's not just about feeling better emotionally: a supportive group of friends and colleagues can help you live a better, healthier life. Having people who care about you significantly reduces stress and makes things easier to handle.

Think of your support system as your squad, the people who can give you a hug or talk things through when you're feeling down. They can be family, friends, or even work buddies. It might be difficult to explain what you're going through during menopause, but it's really important. Your loved ones may not understand why you're experiencing all these changes. Sharing with them can make a huge difference. But how do you share feelings when you barely even understand what you are going through?

Here are some tips for talking to your support system about menopause:

- **Be Honest And Open**: If you don't feel comfortable talking to your support system about menopause, that's understandable. But aim to be honest and open with them about how you're feeling. Talk about what's been going on in your life and why you think it might be due to menopause.

- **Be Specific:** When describing the changes your body is going through, try to use specific language. Explain the symptoms like hot flashes or fluctuating hormones in a way they'll understand.
- **Seek Advice:** Ask for advice on ways to manage stress during menopause or where to find helpful resources. Your general physician would be a useful starting point, but psychologists, counselors, and psychiatrists also cover this ground professionally, so don't be squeamish about asking for professional help when you need it. Menopause societies in your country or state will also have useful advice and where to go for more in-depth information.
- **Be Proactive:** Don't wait until symptoms become overwhelming. Reach out to the people before then and let them know what's happening. They may be able to help you pinpoint what you are feeling too!
- **Join A Support Group:** If you want to maintain your privacy, there are loads of support groups online where you can participate anonymously. Many women find solace in Facebook groups and other online forums. Proximity isn't a factor if you join an online group, but many community organizations provide face-to-face support groups that can bring friendship, comfort, solace and good advice.

Also, don't blame yourself for feeling this way. It's not your fault. Feeling guilty only adds more pressure, and that's definitely not what you need. Finding ways to relieve stress can be very helpful. But if things become too intense, it may be time to talk to your doctor. Sometimes, adjusting your medication or treatment can make a difference. Just remember, your doctor is also there to support you.

I was upfront about my "squad" in my Introduction at the beginning of this book. Two crucial pillars of my sustained optimism and resilience are my Jungian analyst and the hypnotherapist I see when I can't reach things in my conscious mind. I feel no shame (in fact, the opposite) for having regular sessions with these professionals. I confess I can't do all the emotional heavy lifting on my own, and their help and support make a quantum difference in my life. I encourage you to look for your own support, and don't worry if you don't find the right people straight away. It took me many years to settle on what works for me.

If you think you're losing it, I can assure you that you're not! Much of what you're going through is just your body and hormones having a moment. And let's be optimistic; in a few years, you might be the one offering wisdom to another woman or recommending this book. Until then, I want you to repeat the affirmation that you are enough and this, too, shall pass.

But emotional well-being is only one part of the full menopause picture. Next, we'll explore the intimate aspects of relationships during this period of change. Ready to rekindle the flames of intimacy in your life? Stay tuned for Chapter 7.

Chapter 7

Rekindling The Flames of Intimacy

AVRIL'S MENOPAUSE BEGAN with an unwelcome and common problem. She dealt with unexpected and intense emotional struggles – depression and panic attacks.

Sure, these challenges caught her by surprise. But it was a symptom that came in her late 40s that upset Avril the most – she lost her once-strong desire for intimacy. Determined to solve the mystery, Avril consulted a menopause specialist. In this meeting, she discovered the cause of her distress and found a way to deal with it.

So, what exactly happened in Avril's journey?

Before the start of her perimenopause, Avril had been the one who initiated and enjoyed intimacy and physical contact with her partner. But at the start of her menopausal journey, she found her drive for these activities had suddenly plummeted. Her sudden lack of interest was confusing and frustrating, not only for Avril but also for her partner. She felt like a completely different person – one who no longer wanted intimacy or affection.

To gain insight, we need to understand Female Sexual Dysfunction (FSD), which is formally categorized into four aspects: desire, arousal, orgasm, and pain. Research shows that a staggering 30-50 percent of women in the perimenopausal and postmenopausal stages experience sexual difficulties in one or more of these areas.

The Dynamics Of Desire

According to renowned sex educator and psychotherapist Esther Perel, "Eroticism in the home requires active engagement and willful intent." But what happens when you lose the intent and actually want to run in the opposite direction when it is brought up?

Libido is never easy to talk about. Not having sexual desire is difficult enough, but having to discuss this with anyone, let alone your partner, is the cherry on top of the menopausal cataclysm. Let's get this straight: even though the topic is awkward, it's necessary.

However, before your partner can comprehend the changes in your body, you must understand them first. This is a key message here. If you want control over your symptoms, you must understand their cause. Perimenopausal women commonly experience more distressing sexual problems than postmenopausal women even though changes in libido, vaginal dryness, and difficulty reaching orgasm are more common in the latter.

What does that mean? Well, think of it as the difference between a hurricane and the aftermath. The initial storm brings rain, thunder, and lightning that you can't control but can end instantly. The aftermath is when things start to dry up, and what's left behind is in ruins. The first crack of thunder is what people feel when their libido nosedives and everything that comes later is the aftermath.

This loss of libido is one of the most distressing symptoms because you no longer want to initiate or take part in sexual activities. You may not even have any sexual thoughts, and you may have ceased to masturbate. Unfortunately, 50 percent of women in perimenopause and menopause report a decrease in sexual interest or desire. This sheds a doubtful light on your attraction to your partner, the future of your relationship, and most importantly, the quality of your life. I recently heard a women's health doctor on social media speculate that at least half of her menopausal patients get divorced because they can no longer function properly in the bedroom. OK, anecdotal evidence, but if it's true, it's a sad state of affairs, especially when there's effective treatment available.

During menopause, there are three factors that can decrease sexual desire in women: hormonal changes, physical issues, and emotional elements. The main culprit is hormonal changes, specifically the decrease in estrogen levels. This hormonal decline leads to a decrease in libido, unlike during ovulation when estrogen levels are at their highest. On top of that, physical symptoms like fatigue, vaginal dryness, and pain during sex can also contribute to a diminished sex drive.

Arousal is when your body prepares for sex – blood flow increases to the vagina, which becomes lubricated, and breathing and heart rate accelerate. Typically, sexual desire precedes arousal, but as women age and experience menopause, desire and pleasure may occur only *after* arousal. What that means, for example, is that when your partner tries to seduce you or drops hints, you respond with, "Okay, I'm game." Only to discover that the mind may be willing, but the vagina isn't getting the message. Bummer huh?

About 17 to 45 percent of postmenopausal women experience painful sex. It's largely been blamed on vaginal dryness, another common problem during menopause, affecting sexual desire. Lower estrogen levels reduce blood supply to the vagina, causing thinning of vaginal mucosa or atrophy.

This can lead to discomfort or pain during intercourse.

Vaginal dryness can also lead to desensitization, making it harder to orgasm. The clitoris, with its many nerve endings, is vital for female pleasure. Menopause and aging can lower clitoral sensitivity, resulting in longer or less intense orgasms. This condition, known as female orgasmic disorder, is more common in women older than 45.

But other than sexual disorders, vaginal dryness can also cause something a lot more insidious called genitourinary syndrome of menopause (GSM). What is it? Well, it is not just the vagina that loses moisture due to declining estrogen levels. Often, the bladder and the urethra get involved too. This can cause burning, itching, and pain when using the restroom. It also increases the risk of urinary tract infections (UTIs), which can have serious complications if left untreated. In fact, UTIs make up 25 percent of all infections in people over 50.

As someone who has experienced GSM firsthand, I can tell you it's no picnic. Imagine sitting at your desk, minding your own business, and your vagina is saying, "Hello, remember me, I'm in pain. Do something about it, STAT."

Fortunately, GSM has good treatment options but **must** be medically treated. Don't just think it will just go away on its own; it needs hormonal helpers in the form of creams, gels, pills, and other interventions to be controlled. In some cases, vaginal creams will be necessary for the rest of your days.

In the end, when sexual activity becomes unenjoyable and sometimes painful, motivation decreases. Women may find themselves avoiding sex altogether, which can have a negative effect on their relationships with partners.

Physical And Psychological Sparks

In order to ensure a healthy sex life for women, it is important to pay attention to both physical and psychological needs. Physical sparks come from a combination of good circulation, lubrication, hormone balance, and adequate stimulation. Psychological sparks depend on communication with your partner, understanding your body's response to touch and comfort level at that moment. Ensuring you are relaxed will help each component fall into place.

Let's take Jen, who was at her wits end during menopause. She could not sleep, waking up in a pool of sweat multiple times a night. She was tired, experienced brain fog while working, and felt irritable. When her partner tried to have sex with her, she felt like punching her because it felt like one more demand.

And when you're continually exhausted, the last thing you want is one more demand.

The solution to Jen's problem came from fixing one of the root causes of her exhaustion – her inability to sleep properly, which was keeping her exhausted all the time. A Professor of Obstetrics and Gynecology and Director of the Menopause and Sexual Medicine Program at the Center for Women's Health at Oregon Health & Science University (OHSU), Dr. Karen Adams said, "What are those two things that predict a great quality of life? Good sleep and good sex."

But if you don't have the former, the latter can easily be compromised, especially during menopause.

First things first, let's prioritize a good night's sleep. You might be prescribed estrogen to alleviate night sweats and hot flashes. Additionally, we discussed other strategies for better sleep in Chapter 5: adjust the thermostat, remove screens from the bedroom, use blackout curtains, establish a consistent wake-up time, and only go to bed when sleepy. If you can't fall asleep after 20 to 30 minutes, get up and relax in a cozy spot until you feel drowsy, then return to bed.

So, if we get sleep sorted, the next thing to manage is vaginal dryness. GSM is the worst version of it. But here's an alarming statistic: for every two women, one experiences pain during sex after menopause, and only one in twenty seeks treatment. This doesn't have to be your new normal. Don't think your best years of sex are gone by 50. Estrogen is crucial for the vagina, especially to decrease dryness. There are treatment options for you to consider, like vaginal dehydroepiandrosterone (DHEA), low-dose vaginal estrogen rings, and an oral pill option called ospemifene (Osphena).

Sometimes, the pill, patch, or gel you're using may not be enough to keep your vagina comfortable. That's where estrogen cream comes in. The general rule is to apply it every night.

Also, remember to use moisturizers and lubricants. Moisturizers make the vagina plumper and moister when used three times a week, while lubricants during sex can help enormously. It's a good idea to ditch soap in favor of washes that are specifically formulated for your lady parts and contain zero soaps, dyes, parabens, and sulphates.

Let me be clear – using lubricants does not mean you are old. Sixty percent of 20-year-olds use lubricants, so don't think it's only for older women.

It will take some time, but replenishing the estrogen in your body and keeping it moist will help you manage menopause more comfortably and confidently! With quality estrogen cream, lubricants, and moisturizers, you can make sure your best years are ahead of you, not behind you. My call to you is to embrace this new stage of life with grace, dignity and, above all, enthusiasm. But don't suffer in silence; get the help you need, and take the power and pleasure back – so you can enjoy sex and delight in your body.

Now that we have discussed the sparks that can be rekindled physically, let's move on to the emotional and psychological aspects of sex after menopause and how to keep the flame of romance burning even after the hormonal changes that occur during menopause.

Reclaiming Romance

A healthy sex life needs time and attention, and it's easy to let it take a backseat to other important things. Surprisingly, menopause can be a time for rediscovering and renewing romance.

Despite the many physical and emotional differences, one thing remains certain: communication is vital in any relationship. Take the time to discuss your feelings with your partner openly and honestly. If you don't feel comfortable talking about sex directly, discussing related topics like pleasure or romance can be a good starting point. Both of you need to understand each other's needs and expectations to ensure both parties are satisfied.

Rediscovering Emotional Intimacy

What initially attracted you to your partner? Take a trip down memory lane to revive those past feelings and rediscover what is still possible. Recall moments of laughter and shared music to invigorate your emotional intimacy and bring back positive feelings. This will help you rekindle the spark in your relationship.

Reviving Reciprocal Needs

Mutual needs include safety and security, giving and receiving attention, feeling valued and important, and being known and understood. While these needs are non-negotiable, we can discuss the boundaries and limits on how we meet them with each other.

Couples may withdraw from each other when their needs go unmet, resulting in a standoff where both parties are unwilling to take a step forward and restore what has been eroded. Instead, let's adopt an approach of honest inquiry and curiosity to pave the way forward.

Now is the time to explore what you need to feel connected, loved, and safe. Let's start by asking some questions:

What are your requirements?
What are the requirements of your partner?
What are your sexual fantasies?
What does your partner fantasize about?
Is your partner a top priority?
Do both of you feel respected and valued?
What needs to occur for both of you to feel that these needs are being fulfilled?

Our core emotional needs drive us as humans, and successful relationships rely on satisfying these needs mutually. Feeling disconnected in terms of emotional intimacy often stems from a lack of understanding in fulfilling our own or each other's needs in a healthy and sustainable manner.

My hot tip here is to have a play with sex therapist Esther Perel's card game "Where Should We Begin" prompt and story cards, which can really help fire up your intimate conversations.

Finding The Positives

Emotional closeness in a relationship depends on your focus and attention. It's easy to start seeing your partner through a critical lens when you are stressed. To strengthen your bond, create moments of appreciation and acknowledge your partner's efforts to connect. Notice even the smallest positive actions and offer genuine compliments. This will foster emotional connection and cultivate togetherness. Remember, there's always something to appreciate, even when there are things we don't like.

Spice Up Your Relationship

The monotony of a domestic routine can dull intimacy, so it's crucial to be mindful of how you enrich your relationship. Establishing rituals offers a chance to do just that.

Rituals are recurring ways of connecting with each other, infused with a positive emotional element that sets them apart from mere routines. They might be small gestures, but their cumulative impact is powerful.

So, try incorporating gentle rituals into your daily routine. Some ideas include leaving love notes or sending flirty texts, prioritizing being present for each other by greeting each other properly every day and having connecting conversations instead of just problem-solving.

Holistic Healing For Intimacy And Mediating Menopausal Symptoms

Aromatherapy

A fun and intimate date could be to explore essential oils together. Aromatherapy has been used for centuries to reduce stress, anxiety, and even pain. The soothing scents can help you both relax while enjoying time together. To make your own personalized blend, use a carrier oil like jojoba or coconut oil as a base and add three to five drops of your favorite essential oils. Not only is aromatherapy calming, but it can also help regulate hormones responsible for libido within the body.

Essential oils like clary sage, peppermint, lavender, geranium, basil, and citrus have shown promise in alleviating menopause-related discomfort and, when used in a bath or massage, can elevate the experience and bring much-needed intimacy and pleasure.

- **Clary Sage:** Known to mitigate hot flashes when applied to the neck or feet, it may also assist in combating osteoporosis.
- **Peppermint Oil:** Helps relieve hot flashes and menstrual cramping. Caution should be taken if experiencing cramping post-menopause.
- Lavender: Balances hormones, soothes perineal discomfort, aids relaxation, and promotes sleep quality.
- **Geranium:** Provides stress relief, helps with dry skin, and potentially offers antianxiety and antidepressant effects.
- **Basil:** May assist in mood improvement and estrogen level management. Applied to the feet or neck, it can help combat hot flashes.
- **Citrus:** Known to help decrease menopausal symptoms, boost sexual desire, and possess anti-inflammatory properties, citrus essential oils can uplift the mood and boost feelings of well-being. Caution should be exercised as it can sensitize skin to sunlight.

When integrating these treatments into your menopause management, it's essential to consult with certified practitioners and adhere to proper usage instructions.

Herbal Supplements

For natural increases in sex drive, consider adding herbal supplements to your wellness routine. Certain herbs contain properties that can act as aphrodisiacs, increase libido and help manage hormone levels. Examples of herbs that are known for their effectiveness in managing menopause symptoms include:

- **Maca Root:** Helps balance hormones and may reduce symptoms such as hot flashes and vaginal dryness. It also boosts energy, endurance, and stamina. A 2015 study with 45 women who had antidepressant-induced sexual dysfunction showed that taking 3,000 mg of maca root daily for 12 weeks significantly improved sexual function and libido compared to a placebo.
- **Tongkat Ali:** Sometimes known as Longjack, has shown promise in research as a way to boost testosterone levels. Plus, it may have some antidepressant-like properties that can help with mood swings caused by menopause. For sexual health and libido, taking a daily dose of 200–400 mg seems to do the trick. You can split it into two doses per day.
- **Ashwagandha:** Possesses anti-inflammatory properties which can assist with skin health, while potentially offering antianxiety and antidepressant effects. In essence, it is a stress reliever, and that is why it can help with low libido.

Whether you choose herbal supplements or topical treatments, please consult with your doctor before making any decisions. Your doctor can ensure that the supplement or topical treatment is right for you and won't interact with your existing medications.

Remember, the sizzle of sexual attraction may fluctuate, but friendship, respect, fun, and loving intention can help maintain a strong bond. Get creative, put your imagination into finding new ways for intimacy and fun, and reclaim that loving and sensual feeling.

Finally, don't waste time wishing for your sex life back just for someone else's happiness. Your sex drive is about you—it's a vital part of your quality of life. So, don't feel guilty about what you're not giving someone else. Instead, focus on connecting with what you truly need.

So far, we've covered the emotional and physical aspects of menopause. Now, it's time to look at the broader picture of rejuvenation. From the top of your head to the soles of your feet, let's explore how you can feel revitalized in every way. Get ready to embrace rejuvenation from crown to soul in Chapter 8.

Chapter 8

Rejuvenation From Crown To Soul

◆◈─────────────────────────────────────◈◆

PAULA KENNEDY WAS just like many of us during her mid-forties, knowing that it was coming but not knowing what a major transformation it would be.

It was what she saw in the mirror that gave her pause. Everyday.

She was a VP at a London tech firm when the "The Change" started. Always in leadership positions, Paula had the confidence to get through whatever circumstances life presented her. But never before had she faced a challenge like this....

Even while on hormone replacement therapy and taking care of the symptoms as they came up, she still felt "different." In her own words, "For a long time I really grieved the loss of who I used to be (before menopause)."

When Paula looked in the mirror, she saw her mother, which appalled her. Her mother was always overweight when Paula was slim and never even considered dieting. Her once glossy and thick hair had become thin and limp, and her skin was the worst of it – her fresh, rosy, youthful complexion had become ruddy and blotchy with new rosacea marks. All she could think when she appraised her appearance was, "Ugh, not me again."

After a lot of soul-searching, she realized her low mood had more to do with her external transformation than what was going on internally – which was being taken care of with medications.

With a fresh outlook and determination to explore the change, Paula decided to take control of the situation. With the help of a counselor, she stopped judging herself and her appearance and embraced the grace and style that had always been an intrinsic part of how she presented herself. She opted for a new wardrobe, tried different hairstyles and colors, and found her way back to vibrant health.

It took guts and gusto. But in doing so, Paula was able to reclaim her identity and rediscover her self-confidence. As it turns out, transitioning into menopause doesn't have to be daunting – with the right attitude and approach, anyone can find their groove again!

In a society that largely determines value based on appearance, aging women often find themselves at the mercy of rapidly changing fashions and an inability to reconcile what they see in the mirror and who they were before the change.

I could scream with rage at how society devalues older women, making them feel invisible and worthless. One of my main motivators in writing this book was to use my experience as a health and beauty editor to blow up the stereotypes about aging women and empower you to make small changes to your appearance for maximal effect.

This chapter is about holistic rejuvenation – taking care of your external self as you navigate menopause. While it is impossible to turn back the clock, there are ways to help you feel as good on the outside as you're working to feel on the inside. The power is in your hands.

There's so much energy, vitality, and joy to claim when you accept where you are in your journey and embrace the change with the wisdom of an elder. After all, you've only got one life to live – you may as well live it to the fullest.

The Skin-Deep Beauty
And How To Reclaim It

As Betty Friedan said, "Aging is not lost youth, but a new stage of opportunity and strength," and that's no truer than when it comes to taking care of yourself during menopause.

Our skin is the largest organ, and changing hormones can significantly impact it. The hormonal changes can wreak havoc with your skin, especially during perimenopause. In a survey of 87 women attending a specialist menopause clinic, more than 64 percent reported skin problems. This includes having itchy, dry, and thinning skin.

Why does it happen? Well, it's all about the decrease in estrogen levels, which occurs naturally during menopause. When you have lower levels of this key hormone, your body produces less sebum (oil) and collagen than usual. As a result, your skin can become dry, brittle, and thin with more visible wrinkles.

Dry skin can be debilitating, occurring anywhere, such as the corners of your mouth or the sides of your nails. It can cause significant pain, affecting your hands in general and leading to cracked and sore fingertips. Dryness and dehydration are often the culprits behind these issues, including dry heels.

To tackle this issue, look for skincare products with ingredients that help retain moisture. Some ingredients to keep an eye out for are hyaluronic acid, glycerin, and ceramides. This isn't about vanity; it's about wellness, so if you're skeptical about using cosmetics, mistrust the marketing machine that is the modern beauty industry, seriously, think again. A recent study done in 2021 with 40 women aged 30-65 found that using a topical serum with hyaluronic acid can effectively hydrate the skin. Another study from 2017, which involved women with an average age of 40, showed that a product containing hyaluronic acid, glycerin, and centella asiatica (also known as gotu kola) significantly improved skin hydration for a whole 24 hours. So, there are definite steps you can take when looking for the right moisturizer for your skin.

As if feeling like a dried-out prune was not enough, you might also get the added bonus of a resurgence of teenage acne. If you're dealing with acne in menopause, don't worry; help is at hand!

One solution is to try cleansers with salicylic acid or glycolic acid, which gently exfoliate the skin. However, keep in mind that these ingredients may not be suitable for everyone, especially if you have drier than average skin. In that case, using a gentle cleanser might be a better option. Another helpful ingredient is retinol, which can be beneficial if you don't have dry skin. But remember, retinol can make your skin more sensitive to UV rays, so always wear sunscreen, regardless of the weather or season. In fact, everyone should wear daily sunscreen to protect the skin from sun damage and skin cancer!

According to a 2019 review, chemical peels containing ingredients like salicylic acid, glycolic acid, mandelic acid, and retinol can help reduce acne. Combination peels, such as salicylic-mandelic acid in a gel base or lactic acid peels, may be particularly beneficial for those with sensitive maturing skin.

You might also suddenly find yourself sunburned after 15 minutes outside. You might even get discoloration on the skin, like dark patches, or if you have dark skin, you can end up with light patches. Rashes, itchy lumps, and bumps may occur, along with slow wound healing.

That's not all, though. There are so many skin conditions that might not be directly caused by menopause, but their incidence increases for women at this time. Rosacea, for example, is something that usually comes with age, and it's very common in pre and perimenopausal women.

Warts and verruca can also occur when the skin becomes thinner and more susceptible to attacks from various sources. Our immune system may weaken as we age, making it easier for viruses to take hold. These viral infections can be transmitted from other people and surfaces, making them quite common. Be aware of this and take precautions to avoid picking them up unintentionally.

For the immune system and skincare, vitamin C and zinc are excellent for helping maintain skin health.

Moles can also occur due to thinner skin, which can be more sensitive to sun exposure. The skin has a compound called melanin that protects against sunburn. So, when estrogen levels drop, less melanin is produced, which might lead to more moles as we age. Keep an eye on any moles, especially if new ones pop up or if they have weird shapes, because they can turn into skin cancer or be signals for it. If you notice anything strange with your moles, make sure to talk to your doctor. Whilst it's good to get some sunlight for vitamin D, as I said above, don't forget to use sunscreen to protect your skin when you're outside.

Finally, let's talk about the dreaded peach "fuzz." During menopause, a decrease in estrogen can lead to increased hair growth on the face and body. While this is common and natural after menopause, treatments like laser hair removal or waxing can reduce its appearance and help keep your skin looking smooth and youthful.

Ultimately, it doesn't matter what age you are; if you care for your skin as you would for a baby, tending to it with compassion and love, it will reward you with increased radiance and clarity. Confidence comes not just from beauty but also from good self-care, and when it comes to menopause skin care, a little extra effort can go a long way. Self-care is one of the most powerful ways to promote self-love and self-acceptance, so make sure you have an up-to-date skincare routine tailored to your needs, eat right, get plenty of rest, find ways to relax and reduce stress levels, and don't forget to talk to your doctor.

The Mane Event For Hair Care

For Sophie Jones, menopause came with an awful surprise – hair loss. The texture of her hair changed in terms of how thin it felt. Not only did it seem her hair was thinning, especially on the crown, but the strands were breaking, and her hairbrush was full every morning.

She felt her scalp dry up, and the urge to scratch it was almost unbearable. But she knew that scratching her scalp would only make matters worse. After sitting in the chair at her hairdresser and bawling her eyes out she did what everyone tells you to do after 50 to escape this.

Chop it all off!

But this just made her more miserable. Her waist was swelling in size, while her locks, which had been long and shiny with minimal care once, had to be sheared and ended up making her think she looked like a beach ball with a crop on top. How was that fair?

And it's unfair because for so many of us our hair has been our crowning glory and a key to healthy self-esteem. A good hair day and a bad hair day can be the difference between a great day and a decidedly terrible day. It can wreck our confidence. It can even affect how we interact with other people. If we think our hair's an absolute mess, then we're going to be reserved rather than outgoing.

So why does this happen?

Again, it comes back to the tanking level of estrogen. Decreased estrogen levels can impact hair growth in various ways. It can lead to hair thinning, slower growth, and shrinkage of hair follicles. As a result, hair becomes thinner, more brittle, and prone to falling out easily. By age 50, more than half of all women experience this phenomenon. And once they hit 60, an astonishing 80 percent of women are affected by it.

Apart from hormones, nutrition also plays a role. When we go through menopause, our nutritional requirements increase because of those physical changes happening inside. Our body takes in the nutrition it needs to tackle vital matters. And you know what? When we don't get good enough nutrition, our hair is usually the first to feel the effects. Because even if it feels vital to us, our body has different ideas.

This is why our hair is very often a good indication of what the rest of the body needs. Stress can take a toll on us physically and emotionally during this time, burning up essential nutrients. Consequently, our hair may suffer due to a decreased availability of nutrients. Other health issues like low thyroid function or iron deficiency can also significantly affect our hair, particularly if heavy and frequent bleeds occur during perimenopause. So, what should you be on the lookout for?

- Increased hair loss and the need to clean your brush more frequently.
- Noticing more hair on your comb regularly.
- Finding more hair trapped in the shower drain.
- Seeing more hair on your pillow or clothes.
- Picking up more hair while cleaning.
- Thinning ponytail or hair that breaks off easily.
- Difficulty regaining previous hair length.
- Experiencing more split ends.
- Wider parting, revealing more scalp, especially for those with dark hair.
- Thinning at the back of the head and around the temples.
- Lack of body in the hair compared to before.

It seems very simple, but most of us have difficulty paying attention to these nuances and only become aware when it gets too much. Taking action early is important if you're noticing any of these signs.

But here's what you're wondering: will this hair loss stick around for good? You see, with menopause, some symptoms tend to fade away as time goes on. The tricky part about hair loss is that if your nutritional needs are through the roof and you're not meeting them, it's no surprise that this problem won't magically go away.

The key – be proactive. As soon as you notice any signs, that's your cue to step in and prevent things from getting worse. Here are some tips to keep that mane of yours around for as long as possible:

- Make sure you're getting enough protein in your diet – this will help keep your hair strong and promote healthy growth.
- Increase iron intake to ensure your body receives enough nutrients from food.

- Add supplements such as biotin, zinc, and omega-3 fatty acids to your daily routine. These can all help support hair health.
- Revamp your hair-care routine. Acknowledge that your long-standing routine won't do the trick anymore. Seek out products with higher humectant content and increased hydration.
- Use silk, satin, or sateen pillowcases to prevent hair tangling while you sleep, especially for restless sleepers. And use silk scrunchies to tie your hair instead of elastic scrunchies.
- Use dry/wet brushes when shampooing and conditioning to brush through your hair gently. It ensures even product distribution from root to tip.

By following these tips, you'll be able to maintain healthy hair that looks and feels great. Remember, the work you put in your hair today will lead to better hair health in the future.

And, if the worst happens and you do lose a noticeable amount of hair, there are more solutions today than ever before. As the famous comedienne Joan Rivers said, "Looking 50 is great – if you're 60". You certainly don't have to look 60 at 50. Rivers knew all about it. She had her own range of wigs and hair pieces, and on her TV show *Fashion Police*, she often outed herself as a wig-wearer, plastic surgery devotee, and a woman not afraid to use whatever was at her disposal to look her best. You may be surprised to know how many celebrities regularly wear wigs and hairpieces. Lady Gaga, Rihanna, Katy Perry, Zendaya, and Emily Ratajkowski, to name a few, are all women who play with wigs, and thankfully, the stigma of these hair enhancers is a thing of the past.

Today, you can buy hair extensions, halos (which are a kind of headband with hair attached), toppers (mini wigs or wiglets designed to cover a thinning crown) and tapes, which can be attached with clips and weaves (which are actually sewn or glued into the hair) Don't be afraid to try any or all of them. I've tried them all (except full wigs and weaves), and they can give you a much-needed pep for a party or special occasion.

My other great beauty tip is using a hair powder with natural hair fibers to cover up balding patches. There are quite a few on the market, and the idea is that they fill in the gaps with a fluffy cotton powder, which gives the appearance of growing hair. It's a great camouflage and certainly much cheaper than a hairpiece.

Radiant Style To Reflect Your Spirit

The inevitable truth is that your body is evolving as the years go by. Does it feel overwhelming? Yes. Do you want to rip out your "remaining" hair? Probably. Do you want to bury your expanding waist in layers and layers of clothing? Definitely.

But does that mean hating what you see in the mirror? No way!

Undoubtedly, your body's changing shape and size can be hard to accept, but it doesn't have to mean that you don't love yourself. You need to find ways to channel your own unique style – a look that works for your body type flatters your face shape and reflects the resplendent spirit within.

By embracing this new version of yourself, you can unlock new possibilities in styling as well as create a renewed sense of confidence. The best part is that you don't have to conform to everyone's beauty standards. Because the right style will not only make you look good but also uplift your spirit.

Let's look at some of the ways you can find the perfect style for yourself:

Start by objectively assessing your body shape and size – the first step in finding a style that looks good on you is understanding what works best with your figure. The lowering of estrogen often leads to expanding waists. To conceal your tummy and feel more confident, opt for high-waisted bottoms. Embrace styles like A-line dresses, skirts, caftans, and empire waist tops that slim your silhouette. V-neck lines are the most flattering choice if you want to divert attention from your midsection.

Pay attention to color theory when selecting garments and makeup – clothing colors have an impact on how we perceive ourselves, so pick colors that complement your skin tone, eye, and hair color.

The general metric is that there are three different skin tones (whether you are black, white, yellow, brown or anything in between). Start by looking at your arm. To help identify the best colors for skin tone and the foundations of your wardrobe, you'll need to determine whether your skin has a warm undertone, a cool undertone, or a neutral undertone. If the veins on your wrist are more blue than green, you have cool-toned skin. If they're greener, your skin is warm-toned. If it's hard to tell, you likely have a neutral skin tone.

One note: it doesn't matter if you have pale, olive or black, brown or yellowish skin – the shades don't determine your skin tone. For example, you can have pale skin with a warm complexion or black skin with a cool complexion.

If you have cool undertones, go for greys, browns, blues, greens and purples. Avoid soft pastels shades or vivid bright colours. This applies to both clothes and makeup.

If your skin tends to tan rather than burn in the sun, you'll most likely have warm undertones. If your veins are greenish rather than bluish, that's another sign, so is having an olive complexion.

While you generally have a wider color palette to play with, shades that are a bit brighter or darker than the middle range will probably be most flattering. What does that mean, you're asking? A good rule of thumb is to go for pale beige rather than a sandy hue at one end of the color spectrum, and navy rather than pale blue at the other end. Avoid greenish or yellowish shades, which can wash you out, and if you want to go all white or all black, add a splash of color like red or purple. And this goes for makeup as well as clothes.

You're most likely neutral skin-toned if you see both a blue and green tone in your veins. Neutral skin-toned people have a broad range of colors at their disposal. The only color that is usually not flattering for a neutral-toned complexion is yellow. Pastels and brights are both safe for this skin tone, and bright red, orange, or beige and white can flatter individuals with this colored skin.

Fabrics matter. When it comes to comfort, natural fabrics like cotton, linen, and bamboo are usually the way to go. They allow your skin to breathe and keep you feeling fresh. You can also consider cotton-poly blends with a small amount of polyester, as polyester is moisture-wicking and can help keep you dry when you're sweating. However, most synthetic fibers don't breathe well or wick moisture, so they might not be the best choice. Silk is lightweight and breathable, but it doesn't wick moisture and can retain odor, so it's better to wear it as an outer layer if you sweat a lot.

Avoid too-tight clothes – I know you want to push everything that's coming out back in. But it is never that simple. Not only does wearing snug clothing make you feel hot and sweat more, but it can also affect your confidence if you're carrying extra menopause weight. Plus, high necklines tend to trap heat and restrict air circulation.

Caftans are chic, but avoid tents – just because you might steer clear of wearing tight clothes doesn't mean you get to wear a shapeless garbage bag that makes you look like you're hiding under a tarpaulin. Always try to balance baggy pieces without trying to hide your silhouette completely. For example, if you are wearing loose high-waisted trousers, pair them with a figure-skimming top to balance the look. Or if you're wearing a loose dress, add a belt and actually emphasize your waist, even if it's not the cinched-in waist of your youth.

Layers are your best friend – it's all about having easy-to-remove layers that can stand alone, especially for those pesky hot flashes. You don't want to feel too exposed when taking off a top layer. So, think of bra-friendly tanks and tees, and lightweight third layers. Oh, and a light linen scarf can be a lifesaver for quick removal during a hot flash. Just wrap it around your shoulders when the chills kick in.

Now that you know the basics of dressing for hot flashes, it's time to have fun with your wardrobe! Take advantage of the time you feel energized and pick out pieces you love. With clothing items like breezy dresses, high-waisted trousers, and even chunky sweaters, you can create a fashion-forward look while keeping the comfort level up during those uncomfortable moments. Just keep in mind that what you see in the mirror should make you feel confident and empowered.

As Stacy London from the TV show *What Not to Wear* always said, "Step away from the mirror and really look for your reflection elsewhere in the eyes of the people who love and adore you." So, as you embrace this new kind of fashion, remember to own it and always rock the look with confidence!

In the end, even if it doesn't seem like it, you are in control of a lot of things that can bring positive change in your life. Your skin, hair, and style are just some of them, but the most important is how you choose to express yourself. This will allow you to embrace "The Change" with open arms and will help you feel more empowered – from the inside out.

We've covered a lot of ground, from understanding the science behind menopause to taking control of your emotional and physical well-being. As we move into the conclusion, we'll reflect on how you can bring all these elements together for a fulfilling and vibrant life post-menopause.

Conclusion

MY JOURNEY WITH you ends here, but your path towards understanding menopause and embracing it with confidence is just beginning. Because, despite what people will have you believe, it isn't the end; it's a second act, a new start, a reboot and rebirth – a phase full of opportunities to thrive and embrace new potentials.

We started off by understanding the hormonal shifts occurring within the body. And what it means to have this inevitability creep up on you. What kind of tests will you will need to find answers, and how can you keep track of your body's metamorphosis?

When it comes to weight gain during menopause, we've dug deeper into the hormonal changes. But here's the good news: managing your weight doesn't have to be a daunting challenge. By busting the myth of inevitable weight gain, we explored how intermittent fasting blended with nutrient-rich foods can be a helpful tool for staying healthy. We also explored the importance of making mindful nutritional choices and staying active. These strategies can help counter the changes that come with menopause and keep you feeling good overall.

But it's not just about the physical changes. We also addressed the emotional swings and provided guidance for navigating intimate relationships. We can achieve emotional balance and maintain closeness by equipping ourselves with these tools.

Lastly, we embraced this phase of life as a time for reinvention and new beginnings. From skincare and haircare to levelling up your wardrobe, we discussed ways to boost confidence and embrace your unique beauty.

With knowledge, understanding, and practical guidance, women can not only survive but thrive through menopause. But, let's not forget, in this grand adventure called menopause, one thing remains abundantly clear: it's an individual journey.

As you've discovered in this book, menopause doesn't have to be a struggle and it's not a disease to be cured. It's a natural phase of life that is more powerfully embraced, rather than resisted. Menopause is not just a change; it's a rise. It's about you reclaiming and expressing everything that is wonderfully, powerfully YOU.

Now, it's your turn.

How has this book transformed your outlook on menopause, and how will you apply these newfound insights in your daily life? Share your thoughts, leave a review, or just let me know how you're feeling – we're in this together.

Bonus Chapter

Equip Your Menopausal Toolkit

YOU HAVE COME to the end of your journey of learning more about your natural clock, but your path towards embracing and owning menopause is just beginning. While each of us has a unique experience of menopause, and let's face it, not all of us will have the same symptoms, the fact remains that we will ALL go through "The Change."

And what is the best way not to be caught off guard and face menopause with confidence? The answer lies in building your very own menopausal toolkit. This includes everything you need to navigate this transition with ease, comfort, and grace.

In this bonus chapter, we will discuss some essential tools to make your menopausal journey smoother and less disastrous.

Menopause Symptom Checker

"The Change" comes with its own set of challenges, and it's essential to understand what your body is going through. So, the first question should always be:

"Is it menopause or something else entirely?"

As a woman who has reached this phase of life and thought herself ready to deal with what's to come, I was still surprised by how much

I didn't know or how certain things are emphasized while others still remain shrouded in mystery.

Don't worry! If you're unsure whether you've reached this stage in your life and questioning if your PMS is simply prolonged, use this comprehensive checklist to determine if it's time to bid farewell to your monthly menstruation and tackle a different beast entirely.

Symptom Checklist

Gut Troubles

- Constipation
- Diarrhea
- Fecal incontinence (which means difficulty controlling your bowels)
- Heartburn or gastric reflux

Breast

- Tender breasts (even a hug hurts)
- Breast growth (going up a size, or two)
- Nipples sensitive to the touch
- Swelling and lumpiness

Heart

- Palpitations and a racing heart, even at rest
- Your chest feels tight or heavy
- Feeling anxious and jittery due to adrenaline surges

Ear, Nose And Throat

- Tinnitus: Ringing in your ears
- Globus sensation: Feeling like something is stuck in your throat
- Voice Changes: Hoarseness or a deeper voice

Eyes

- Dry Eyes (itching and irritation)
- Watery eyes (constantly wiping away tears)

Genital

- Vaginal dryness: Discomfort during activities like intercourse.
- Vaginal discharge: The vagina produces discharge to maintain cleanliness and health. Any changes in color, odor, or consistency may signal an underlying issue.
- Vulval itch: Itching or irritation in the external genital area.
- Perineal itch: Itching in the perineal area, which is the space between the vagina and anus.

Menstrual

- Periods on the rise: more frequent, like a never-ending symphony.
- Longer cycles: less frequent, giving you a break from the crimson tide.
- Heavy periods
- Lighter periods

Metabolic

- Weight gain: You start to feel fatigued, bloated, and your clothes just don't fit like they used to.
- Insulin resistance: Your body becomes less responsive to insulin, leading to an increase in blood sugar levels.
- Fat redistribution: You may notice fat accumulation in certain areas, such as your midsection or face.
- Changes in cholesterol levels: Your body may start producing more LDL (bad) cholesterol and less HDL (good) cholesterol. This is more a sign than a symptom since you will only get to know about this during your blood panels.
- Low tolerance to alcohol: You can no longer hold your liquor like you used to. Your body is struggling to metabolize alcohol, leading to quicker intoxication and hangovers that seem to last forever.

Mood And Cognitive Health

- Crying: Due to a minor inconvenience or even unknown reasons!
- Brain fog: You may find yourself having trouble focusing.
- Memory fog: You open your fridge and forget what you wanted to get.
- Poor concentration: Bye-bye laser focus, hello distraction!
- Word-finding difficulty: It's on the tip of your tongue, but you can't remember that word.
- Anxiety: The stress of daily living is making you more jittery than usual.
- Low mood: You can no longer find joy in anything.
- Worsening PMS: Your PMS symptoms now seem unbearable.
- Anger: The rage at the most minor things is starting to take over.
- Irritability: You find yourself snapping at loved ones for no reason.
- Restlessness: You can't seem to relax, even when you have nothing to do.
- Migraines: The throbbing pain in your head is becoming a regular occurrence.
- Insomnia: You can't seem to fall asleep, no matter how tired you are.
- Fatigue: You are not just tired but exhausted all the time.

Musculoskeletal

- Joint pain: The cracks are starting to hurt now.
- Joint stiffness: It's becoming harder to move without pain.
- Back pain: You can't seem to find a comfortable position anymore.
- Frozen shoulder: Your range of motion is limited and painful.
- Tennis elbow: The pain is becoming persistent and affecting your daily activities.
- Plantar fasciitis: Every step you take feels like a punch to the foot.
- Muscle loss: You feel weaker and less capable of physical activities.
- Restless legs syndrome: Your legs won't stop twitching, making it hard to relax.

Oral

- Burning mouth syndrome: Your mouth feels like it's on fire, even though there's no visible cause.
- Dry mouth: No matter how much water you drink, your mouth still feels dry.
- Tooth decay: You're starting to notice cavities and toothaches more frequently.
- Gum disease: Your gums are swollen, bleeding, and sensitive to touch.

Skin And Hair

- Itchy and dry skin: Moisturizers don't seem enough to treat the dryness, cracking, and itchiness.
- Rosacea: Your face is constantly red and inflamed.
- Hair loss: You're noticing more hair falling out and thinning spots on your scalp.
- Acne: Despite trying different products, your skin is still breaking out.
- Thinning skin: Your skin bruises easily and takes longer to heal.
- Loss of collagen and elasticity in skin.
- Change in pigmentation, such as age spots and dark circles.
- Unwanted hair growth: You're noticing dark, coarse hair in areas such as your chin and upper lip.

Urinary Symptoms

- Infections: You often experience frequent or severe infections, especially after sex.
- Frequency: You have to go more often than usual.
- Urgency: You feel the sudden need to go, like right now.
- Nocturia: You find yourself getting up at night to use the bathroom.
- Incontinence: You struggle with poor control over your bladder.

Vasomotor

- Night sweats: Those unexpected sweaty nights that leave you feeling damp and uncomfortable.
- Hot flashes: Sudden waves of heat that make you feel like you're standing in a sauna, even when everyone else is comfortable.
- Cold flashes: The opposite of hot flashes, these chilling sensations can leave you shivering and reaching for a cozy blanket.
- Raynaud's: A condition where your fingers or toes may turn white or blue in response to cold temperatures or stress, making them feel numb or tingly.

If the symptoms listed above sound familiar and you're struggling to find relief, then you might be the end of an era.... Or at least the beginning of an end. These symptoms can show up in various intensities in different individuals, so remember that just because your friend had hot flashes first does not negate your brain fog, and just because you have cold flashes doesn't mean you won't experience mood swings. If any single symptom or collection of symptoms is causing even mild distress, book in with your doctor and use the symptom checker as a starting point for an honest conversation.

If you need more information about a particular symptom, don't hesitate to review the additional resources listed below. Because educating yourself is the best way to prepare for this inevitability and get clarity on what you might be going through.

- Administration on Aging (AoA), HHS
- Centers for Disease Control and Prevention (CDC), HHS
- Eunice Kennedy Shriver National Institute of Child Health and Human Development (NICHD), NIH, HHS
- Food and Drug Administration (FDA), HHS
- National Institute of Mental Health (NIMH), NIH, HHS
- National Institute on Aging (NIA), NIH, HHS
- American Congress of Obstetricians and Gynecologists
- Hormone Health Network
- North American Menopause Society (NAMS)
- Red Hot Mamas Menopause Support Group

If you're not in the USA, there are menopause societies in most countries you can use as a starting point:

Australia:

- Australasian Menopause Society

Canada:

- Menopause and U Canada
- Canadian Menopause Society

United Kingdom:

- Women's Health Concern
- Menopause Matters

Keeping Score with Your Body

Once you have identified your symptoms and educated yourself through the power of research and the internet, the next step is to get cozy with your body and mind. You need to focus on what's happening.

Easier said than done, I know!

The more you keep score of each symptom, the better you can track your response and progression. By monitoring your own symptoms and reactions, you can collect better data and understand what works for you and what doesn't.

Keep a journal or use a tracking app to record your daily experiences. Take note of any physical changes, emotional fluctuations, and overall well-being. This will not only help you monitor your progress but also provide valuable information when discussing treatment options with your healthcare provider.

When you have an idea of what your treatment is going to be like and which specific symptoms to tackle first, you need to set goals for yourself. These goals should be realistic and achievable, taking into account your current lifestyle and schedule.

For example, if you are experiencing hot flashes, your goal could be to reduce their frequency or intensity within a month. Or if you are struggling with mood swings, your goal could be to find healthy coping mechanisms to manage them within three months. Whatever your goals, make sure they align with your overall well-being and are something you can realistically work towards.

If you're having trouble defining your goal, try using the SMART approach to make it more concrete. SMART stands for Specific, Measurable, Achievable, Relevant, and Time-based. This will turn a goal like, "I want to feel better" into "I will exercise for 30 minutes, three times a week, to improve my energy levels and mood within two months."

If you still find your predicament confusing and would rather seek help from someone who specializes in goal-setting, consider reaching out to a therapist or life coach. They can help you identify your values and priorities and create a personalized plan to reach your goals.

Remember, setting goals is an ongoing process. As you progress towards one goal, don't be afraid to set new or adjust existing ones. And most importantly, be kind to yourself throughout the journey. You may face setbacks or challenges, but every step forward is a victory worth celebrating.

Additionally, it's important to prioritize self-care in your journey towards menopause. This includes taking time for yourself, relaxation techniques such as meditation or yoga, getting enough sleep, and practicing maintaining a healthy diet. It's also key to seek support from loved ones or professionals if you're struggling with any emotional or physical symptoms.

Menopause can be a challenging time, but by setting realistic goals and prioritizing self-care, you can navigate through this transition with more ease and confidence.

If the Symptom Checker left you with some doubts about whether you're in perimenopause, menopause, or post-menopause, take a few minutes to do this easy quiz and use it as a starting point for a chat with your healthcare provider.

Menopause Symptom Quiz #2

Section 1: Physical Symptoms

- **Hot Flashes**

    a) Never
    b) Occasionally
    c) Frequently
    d) Almost daily

- **Night Sweats**

    a) Never
    b) Occasionally
    c) Frequently
    d) Almost every night

- **Irregular Periods**

    a) No change
    b) Mild irregularity
    c) Highly irregular
    d) Periods have stopped completely

- **Vaginal Changes**

    a) No discomfort
    b) Mild discomfort
    c) Moderate discomfort
    d) Severe discomfort and dryness

- **Sleep Disturbances**

    a) No trouble sleeping
    b) Occasionally disrupted sleep
    c) Frequently have trouble falling or staying asleep
    d) Consistent difficulty sleeping

Section 2: Emotional and Mental Health Symptoms

- **Mood Swings**

  a) Rarely experience mood swings
  b) Occasionally feel irritable or anxious
  c) Frequently experience mood swings
  d) Mood swings are a daily occurrence

- **Memory Issues**

  a) No noticeable memory problems
  b) Occasional forgetfulness
  c) Frequent memory lapses
  d) Severe memory problems affecting daily life

- **Changes in Libido**

  a) No change in libido
  b) Slight decrease in interest
  c) Moderate decrease in interest
  d) Significant decrease in interest or no interest at all

- **Emotional Health**

  a) No change in emotional well-being
  b) Occasional feelings of sadness or low mood
  c) Frequent feelings of sadness or low mood
  d) Consistent feelings of depression or lack of motivation

Section 3: Physical Changes

- **Skin and Hair Changes**

  a) No changes
  b) Mild changes in skin or hair texture
  c) Noticeable changes in skin or hair
  d) Significant changes in skin or hair quality

- **Cardiovascular Changes**

    a) No noticeable changes
    b) Occasional heart palpitations or fluctuations in blood pressure
    c) Frequent heart palpitations or fluctuations in blood pressure
    d) Severe cardiovascular changes

- **Digestive Issues**

    a) No digestive issues
    b) Occasional bloating or gas
    c) Frequent bloating, gas, or changes in bowel habits
    d) Severe digestive problems

Scoring

Assign points based on the options chosen:

a)= 0 points
b)= 1 point
c)= 2 points
d)= 3 points

Calculate the total points and interpret as follows:

- 0-10 points: Low likelihood of menopausal symptoms.
- 11-25 points: Moderate likelihood of experiencing menopausal symptoms.
- 26-36 points: Higher likelihood of menopausal symptoms.

Remember, this quiz is not a replacement for professional medical advice. Consult a healthcare provider for an accurate assessment and guidance if you suspect menopausal symptoms.

An Invitation To Share

"I want to build a community where women of all races can communicate and… continue to support and take care of each other. I want to give women a space to feel their own strength and tell their stories. That is power."

- Beyoncé

Dear Reader

You're nearly at the end of my book and I hope you're enjoying reading it as much as I loved writing it.

As you know from my story at the beginning of this book, I've gone through many of the symptoms and challenges you have on your menopause journey. My mission has been to share information and wisdom and empower people like you. Everything I do is aligned with this value.

I'd like to invite you to jump on board with me and my mission to empower people by leaving a review for this book. Your gift won't cost you any money and will take less than 60 seconds of your time, but in giving this gift, you'll be sharing what you've learned with someone else.

A percentage of my profits go to various charities. I'm particularly passionate about ending slavery and supporting Doctors Without Borders.

May the blessings flow to you from this gift of sharing.

Nikki
www.go2gurupublishing.com

Key Chapter
By Chapter Takeaways

Say Hello To Menopause

- Menopause is when you haven't experienced any menstrual bleeding for 12 consecutive months.
- Declining reproductive hormone levels lead to perimenopause symptoms that can last from four to eight years.
- There's no foolproof test to determine if you're perimenopausal, but healthcare professionals can use assessment tools like MENQOL, Kupperman Index, and MRS to evaluate symptoms and quality of life in menopausal women.
- The most accurate test for menopause is a hormone panel that measures FSH and estradiol levels.
- Mood changes like anger and rage can impact you throughout your menopause journey, starting from the earliest signs of perimenopause all the way to post-menopause.

Demystifying The Hormone Changes

- From birth, females possess all their eggs (around one to two million) in an immature state. Hormones trigger monthly ovulation, releasing the most mature egg for potential fertilization.
- Menopause is characterized by erratic ovulation, decreased egg count and quality, fluctuating estrogen levels, and eventual stabilization at lower levels than before.
- HRT means to give hormones back during the estrogen-deficient state. Synthetic hormone replacement therapy includes

variations like ethinyl estradiol, norethindrone, and Premarin derived from pregnant mare urine.

- Recent studies also suggest that starting hormone replacement therapy (HRT) early in menopause may lower the risk of Alzheimer's and dementia.
- Natural alternatives to HRT include dietary supplements like B vitamins, vitamin E, vitamin D, fibre and omega-3s. These supplements may help regulate energy, reduce hot flashes, neutralize oxidative stress, improve bone health, and aid in lubrication.
- Breast cancer mainly affects those over the age of 40 or with a family history of the disease. Early detection is key, and routine screening with mammograms and ultrasounds is recommended. Physical breast exams and self-exams are also important but can't replace more accurate tests. For women with a family history of breast cancer, hormone therapy does not increase the risk of breast cancer.
- Hormone therapy has not been proven to increase the risk of breast cancer.
- Hormone therapy can reduce the risk of broken bones and osteoporosis.
- Hormone therapy can be an effective treatment for hot flashes and night sweats. It can also help improve mood, sleep quality, fatigue and quality of life.
- For women with a uterus (ie they haven't had a hysterectomy) and who take estrogen combined with progesterone, there is no increased risk of uterine cancer.
- For women without a uterus who take estrogen, for the first seven years there is no increased risk or breast cancer. (The risk may increase slightly past seven years).

Move, Groove, And Improve

- During menopause, the loss of estrogen and testosterone can lead to weight gain, inflammation, and fatigue. Age-related muscle loss and a slower metabolism also contribute to decreased energy levels.

- Hormones like insulin, leptin, ghrelin, GLP-1, and cortisol also play a significant role in weight gain.
- Joint pain during menopause is common, with nearly 40 percent of women aged 45-65 experiencing it. Exercise can effectively reduce inflammation and pain.
- By improving strength and balance, exercise can alleviate joint pain and prevent future injury. One of the key suggestions is to lift heavy weights, performing sets of three to five reps with ample rest.
- Aerobic exercises like brisk walking, running, swimming, and cycling can help with weight loss and increase energy levels. Aim for 30 minutes of exercise five days a week or spread it out over shorter periods.
- Pilates and yoga are also effective in improving flexibility, balance, muscle strength, and endurance. Pilates mat exercises offer a great starting point, focusing on core strength, spinal mobility, and flexibility.

Ditch The Weight, Not The Cake

- Intermittent fasting can help maintain hormonal balance during menopause and address conditions like polycystic ovarian syndrome (PCOS). It has also been associated with reduced risk factors for cancer and improved bone health.
- The 16:8 Method, Alternate Day Fasting, 5:2 Diet, and Eat-Stop-Eat are some popular fasting regimens. Stay hydrated with water and avoid calorie-containing drinks.
- The Mediterranean diet is a versatile and healthy option during perimenopause and menopause. It emphasizes antioxidant-rich plant-based foods, incorporating herbs and spices for flavor.
- To incorporate the Mediterranean diet into your routine, increase your vegetable intake, moderate fruit consumption, opt for high-quality red meat, include oily fish, add nuts and seeds, and cut out "white" foods.
- Maintaining a healthy lifestyle involves having nutritious snacks on hand to combat munchies and reduce stress. Dark chocolate,

black and green tea, probiotics, omega-3 fatty acids, and herbal supplements can all help lower cortisol levels.

Into The Tranquil Night

- Around 40 percent of women face sleep problems during late 40s to early 50s, coinciding with menopause.
- Hot flashes and night sweats can cause disrupted sleep, flushed cheeks, and next-day fatigue. Nearly 44 percent of women with severe hot flashes experience insomnia.
- Other problems include sleep-associated breathing and movement disorders such as snoring, sleep apnea, restless legs syndrome, and periodic limb movements disorder. These conditions can disrupt sleep and cause uncomfortable sensations and involuntary movements in the legs.
- CBTI, or cognitive-behavioral therapy for insomnia, is an effective treatment that helps improve sleep quality and reduces symptoms of chronic insomnia. It involves addressing negative thought patterns and working with a therapist to develop personalized strategies for better sleep.
- Optimizing sleep hygiene is crucial for quality rest. Establishing a consistent sleep schedule, following a nightly routine, and creating a soothing sleep environment are key steps to prioritize sleep.
- Tart cherries, kiwi fruit, and walnuts are all foods that promote sleep. Consuming healthy and low-calorie snacks, like Greek yogurt with cocoa powder or sliced apples with nut butter, about an hour before bedtime can help support a stable blood sugar level and promote satiety until morning.

Mood Swings In The Rear View Mirror

- During menopause, the decline in estrogen affects the amygdala, leading to increased reactions and reduced emotional control. Serotonin levels may also decrease, causing mood swings and decreased happiness. Additionally, emotional fluctuations can be influenced by stress, lack of sleep, dehydration, and low blood sugar.

- Menopause can also result in obsessive behaviors and difficulties with memory recall, task focus, and memory retrieval. Heightened fears, including intense worry for loved ones and negative thinking, may also be experienced during this time.
- To improve mood swings, consider using breathing techniques, meditation, and mindfulness training. Practicing deliberate breathing and mindfulness can help create a sense of balance and gratitude in life.
- Start and end your day on a positive note by using affirmations. These can help shape a positive mindset, particularly during mood swings.
- It's also important to be honest and open with your support system about how you're feeling. Use clear, medically-informed language to describe the changes in your body and seek advice on managing stress.

Rekindling The Flames Of Intimacy

- Genitourinary symptoms like pain during sex after menopause are common for many women, but only a small percentage seek treatment.
- Treatment options for managing this issue include vaginal dehydroepiandrosterone (DHEA), low-dose vaginal estrogen rings, and an oral pill called ospemifene (Osphena).
- Estrogen cream can be used to alleviate discomfort and increase flexibility in the vagina. Moisturizers and lubricants are helpful for maintaining vaginal moisture and comfort.
- Communication is vital to maintaining a healthy sex life during menopause, and discussing feelings and needs with your partner is important. Rediscovering emotional intimacy and reviving past positive feelings can help rekindle the spark in a relationship.
- Understanding and meeting each other's needs is crucial for maintaining a strong connection.

Rejuvenation From Crown To Soul

- Menopause can bring about significant changes, both internally and externally.
- Decreased estrogen levels during menopause can lead to dry and thinning skin. To retain moisture, look for skincare products with hyaluronic acid, glycerin, and ceramides. Cleansers with salicylic acid or glycolic acid can help with acne, but be cautious if you have dry skin. Retinol is beneficial, but remember to wear sunscreen for UV protection.
- Pay attention to signs early to prevent hair loss and promote healthy hair. Meet your nutritional needs by ensuring a sufficient intake of protein and iron. Consider supplements like biotin, zinc, and omega-3 fatty acids. Improve your hair-care routine with products high in humectants. Use silk or satin pillowcases and scrunchies to prevent tangling.
- Choose garments that complement your features and prioritize comfort with breathable fabrics. Layer for easy removal and prioritize well-being for a fulfilling post-menopause life.

About The Author

NIKKI GOLDSTEIN IS the author of 11 books and an awarded copywriter and journalist. She began her career at Vogue and went on to hold senior editorial positions at Elle and Marie-Claire. Nikki's well-known for her highly successful GirlForce, a teen girl self-empowerment series of seven books published by ABC/Harper Collins in Australia and Bloomsbury in the USA. *GirlForce* was converted into a brand by Target and sold yoga wear, cosmetics, stationery, and music under the *GirlForce* brand banner. The series was published in the USA, Russia, Israel, and Greece. In 2004 *GirlForce* won a prestigious Australian Publishing Association award, the Random House Best Designed Children's Series.

Nikki is also the author of *Essential Energy – A Guide to Aromatherapy and Essential Oils* which won a New York Book Fair prize for Best Cover, as well as several international art director's awards for design. Cindy Crawford endorsed it on MTV's House of Style as her, "Favorite coffee table book."

With a passion for helping people be their best selves, Nikki has studied counseling and Jungian studies.

When not working on her publishing business Go2Guru, she's attending to her two needy dachshunds, Archie and Sunny or doing yoga on her deck in Sydney.

www.go2gurupublishing.com

References

Introduction

"50 Over 50 2022" https://www.forbes.com/sites/maggiemc-grath/2022/10/06/introducing-the-50-over-50-2022-women-step-ping-into-their-power-in-lifes-second-half/?sh=563ec95d7227

"Facts About Middle Aged Women Retailers Should Know" https://www.forbes.com/sites/jennmcmillen/2022/10/17/6-facts-about-mid-dle-aged-women-retailers-should-know/?sh=2c0cdcd94ef4

Chapter 1

"10 myths about menopause." (n.d.). *Balancehormoneoklahoma.com*. Retrieved December 30, 2023, from https://www.balancehormoneokla-homa.com/blog/10-myths-about-menopause

"A guide to embracing menopause." (n.d.). *Suryaprananutrition.co.uk*. Retrieved December 30, 2023, from https://www.suryaprananutrition.co.uk/blog/a-guide-to-embracing-menopause

Behrman, S., & Crockett, C. (2023). "Severe mental illness and the peri-menopause." *BJPsych Bulletin, 1–7*. https://doi.org/10.1192/bjb.2023.89

BigWing Interactive. (2015, July 22). "Emotions to expect when going through menopause." *Walnuthillobgyn.com*; Walnut Hill OBGYN. https://walnuthillobgyn.com/blog/what-emotions-to-expect-during-menopause/

Byzak, A. (2017, September 7). "Menopause: What to expect and when to seek help." Tri-City Medical Center. https://www.tricitymed.org/2017/09/menopause-expect-seek-help/

"Do I need to see a doctor for menopause?" (2018, September 21). Pacific Gynecology & Obstetrics Medical Group. https://www.pacgyn.com/need-see-doctor-menopause/

"Emotions and the menopause: mood swings, anxiety and depression." (2022, January 11). *Healthtalk.* https://healthtalk.org/menopause/emotions-and-the-menopause-mood-swings-anxiety-and-depression

Gharpure, M. (2021, August 3). "Try a new hobby." *Graceofnoage.com.* https://www.graceofnoage.com/try-a-new-hobby-menopause/

Maza, E. (2016, August 23). "Menopause: A wonderful stage of personal growth." *Exploring Your Mind.* https://exploringyourmind.com/menopause-wonderful-stage-personal-growth/

"Menopause." (2023, May 25). Mayo Clinic. https://www.mayoclinic.org/diseases-conditions/menopause/symptoms-causes/syc-20353397

"Menopause and your mental wellbeing." (2022, November 29). *NHS Inform.* https://www.nhsinform.scot/healthy-living/womens-health/later-years-around-50-years-and-over/menopause-and-post-menopause-health/menopause-and-your-mental-wellbeing/

"Mood changes during perimenopause are real. Here's what to know." (n.d.). *Acog.org.* Retrieved December 30, 2023, from https://www.acog.org/womens-health/experts-and-stories/the-latest/mood-changes-during-perimenopause-are-real-heres-what-to-know

Pietrangelo, A. (2022, September 19). "7 misconceptions about menopause." *Healthline.* https://www.healthline.com/health/menopause/menopause-misconceptions

Pinkerton, J. V. (2021, November 11). "Debunking the most common menopause myths." *MSD Manual Consumer Version; MSD Manuals.* https://www.msdmanuals.com/home/news/editorial/2021/11/09/20/22/ debunking-the-most-common-menopause-myths

"Reinventing self: Giving yourself permission in menopause." (n.d.). *Sonaturellewellness.com.* Retrieved December 30, 2023, from https://www.sonaturellewellness.com/blog/reinventing-self-giving-yourself-permission-in-menopause

Roosevelt, E. (n.d.). A quote from *You Learn by Living. Goodreads. com.* Retrieved December 30, 2023, from https://www.goodreads.com/ quotes/3823-you-gain-strength-courage-and-confidence-by-every-experience-in

Roz. (2023, September 4). "Embracing menopause: A positive journey of self-discovery and empowerment." Total Health and Wellness | MedSpa in Dayton. https://drrozmd.com/menopause/embracing-menopause-a-positive-journey-of-self-discovery-and-empowerment/

"The emotional roller coaster of menopause." (n.d.). *WebMD.* Retrieved December 30, 2023, from https://www.webmd.com/menopause/ emotional-roller-coaster

Valand, S. (2019, August 22). "How journaling can improve menopause symptoms." Samantha Valand. https://samanthavaland.com/ how-journaling-can-improve-menopause-symptoms/

"What is menopause?" (n.d.). National Institute on Aging. Retrieved December 30, 2023, from https://www.nia.nih.gov/health/what-menopause

"When should I Talk To My Doctor About Menopause?" (n.d.). *Awhcare. com.* Retrieved December 30, 2023, from https://www.awhcare.com/ blog/508880-when-should-i-talk-to-my-doctor-about-menopause/

Chapter 2

"Benefits and risks of hormone replacement therapy (HRT)." (n.d.). *Nhs.uk*. Retrieved December 30, 2023, from https://www.nhs.uk/medicines/hormone-replacement-therapy-hrt/benefits-and-risks-of-hormone-replacement-therapy-hrt/

Bezzant, N. (2022, January 18). "'She will not become dull and unattractive': The charming history of menopause and HRT." *The Guardian*. https://www.theguardian.com/world/2022/jan/18/she-will-not-become-dull-and-unattractive-the-charming-history-of-menopause-and-hrt

"Changes in Hormone Levels." (n.d.). *Menopause.org*. Retrieved December 30, 2023, from https://www.menopause.org/for-women/sexual-health-menopause-online/changes-at-midlife/changes-in-hormone-levels

Cherney, K. (2023, May 9). "Premenopause, perimenopause, and menopause." *Healthline*. https://www.healthline.com/health/menopause/difference-perimenopause

Committee on the Clinical Utility of Treating Patients with Compounded Bioidentical Hormone Replacement Therapy, Board on Health Sciences Policy, Health and Medicine Division, & National Academies of Sciences, Engineering, and Medicine. (2020). "The clinical utility of compounded bioidentical hormone therapy: A review of safety, effectiveness, and use (D. R. Mattison, R. M. Parker, & L. M. Jackson, Eds.)." *National Academies Press*.

"Compounding: Inspections, recalls, and other actions." (2023, December 20). U.S. Food and Drug Administration; FDA. https://www.fda.gov/drugs/human-drug-compounding/compounding-inspections-recalls-and-other-actions

EPOCH. (2021, August 31). "Wicked or wise? Menopausal women in popular history." *Epochmagazine*. https://www.epoch-magazine.com/post/wicked-or-wise-menopausal-women-in-popular-history

Gunter, J. (2023, October 17). "Misinformation about bioidentical and compounded hormones." *The Vajenda*. https://vajenda.substack.com/p/misinformation-about-bioidentical

Harper-Harrison, G., & Shanahan, M. M. (2023). "Hormone Replacement Therapy." *StatPearls Publishing*.

Hill, K. (1996). "The demography of menopause." *Maturitas, 23(2), 113–127.* https://doi.org/10.1016/0378-5122(95)00968-x

"Hormone replacement therapy (HRT)." (n.d.). *Nhs.uk*. Retrieved December 30, 2023, from https://www.nhs.uk/medicines/hormone-replacement-therapy-hrt/

"Hormone replacement therapy (HRT)." (2022, November 3). *NHS Inform*. https://www.nhsinform.scot/tests-and-treatments/medicines-and-medical-aids/types-of-medicine/hormone-replacement-therapy-hrt/

"Hormone therapy: Is it right for you?" (2022, December 6). Mayo Clinic. https://www.mayoclinic.org/diseases-conditions/menopause/in-depth/hormone-therapy/art-20046372

"Hormones." (n.d.). Cleveland Clinic. Retrieved December 30, 2023, from https://my.clevelandclinic.org/health/articles/22464-hormones

"Hot flashes: What can I do?" (n.d.). National Institute on Aging. Retrieved December 30, 2023, from https://www.nia.nih.gov/health/hot-flashes-what-can-i-do

"Is HRT safe for menopause? New guidelines say yes." (2023, February 13). *Uhhospitals.org*. https://www.uhhospitals.org/blog/articles/2023/02/is-hrt-safe-for-menopause-new-guidelines-say-yes

"Is HRT safe to use for the menopause? What the science says." (n.d.). *Ox.ac.uk*. Retrieved December 30, 2023, from https://www.ox.ac.uk/research/hrt-safe-use-menopause-what-science-says-0

Landau, M. D., & Smythe, K. L. (n.d.). "Perimenopause vs. Menopause: A look at the difference." *Everydayhealth.com*. Retrieved December 30, 2023, from https://www.everydayhealth.com/menopause/perimenopause-vs-menopause-look-difference/

Mandal, A., & Sally Robertson, B. S. (2009, November 25). "What are hormones?" *News-medical.net*. https://www.news-medical.net/health/What-are-Hormones.aspx

"Menopause." (n.d.). *Yourhormones.Info*. Retrieved December 30, 2023, from https://www.yourhormones.info/endocrine-conditions/menopause/

"Menopause and weight." (n.d.). *Gov.au*. Retrieved December 30, 2023, from https://www.betterhealth.vic.gov.au/health/conditionsand treatments/menopause-and-weight-gain

"Mood swings during menopause: Causes and treatments." (2017, May 22). *Medicalnewstoday.com*. https://www.medicalnewstoday.com/articles/317566

Ob-Gyn, M. (2022, March 31). "What are the pros and cons of hormone replacement therapy for menopause?" *Morelandobgyn.com*. https://www.morelandobgyn.com/blog/pros-and-cons-of-hormone-replacement-therapy

"Perimenopause." (n.d.). Cleveland Clinic. Retrieved December 30, 2023, from https://my.clevelandclinic.org/health/diseases/21608-perimenopause

"Risk of breast cancer with HRT: progesterone is safer than progestins." (2023). https://www.bmj.com/content/376/bmj.o485/rr-0

Scripps Health. (2022, December 6). "How to tell the difference between perimenopause and menopause." Scripps Health. https://www.scripps.org/news_items/6457-how-to-tell-the-difference-between-perimenopause-and-menopause

Thurrott, S. (n.d.). "The pros and cons of HRT for menopause." *Bannerhealth.com*. Retrieved December 30, 2023, from https://www.bannerhealth.com/healthcareblog/better-me/pros-and-cons-of-hrt-for-menopause-symptoms

Watson, K. (2018, October 26). "36 alternatives to HRT: Diet, supplements, lifestyle changes, and more." *Healthline*. https://www.healthline.com/health/menopause/alternatives-to-hrt

"What you should know about HRT." (n.d.). *WebMD*. Retrieved December 30, 2023, from https://www.webmd.com/menopause/ss/slideshow-hormone-therapy

"What's the difference between perimenopause and menopause?" (n.d.). *Cwcobgyn.com*. Retrieved December 30, 2023, from https://www.cwcobgyn.com/blog/whats-the-difference-between-perimenopause-and-menopause

Chapter 3

Menopause Charity. (2021a, April 24). "Exercise advice." *The Menopause Charity*. https://www.themenopausecharity.org/2021/04/24/exercise-advice/

Menopause Charity. (2021b, June 12). "How can yoga manage your menopause?" *The Menopause Charity*. https://www.themenopausecharity.org/2021/06/12/how-can-yoga-manage-your-menopause/

Albarda, V. (2016, March 14). "Fitness and midlife women: Cardio and strength training." *Midlife-A-Go-Go*; Valerie Albarda. https://www.midlifeagogo.com/fitness-and-midlife-women/

Aliabadi, T. (2015, September 21). "Menopausal joint pain." Dr. Aliabadi, Best Los Angeles OBGYN, Surgeon; Thais Aliabadi, M.D. Los Angeles OBGYN, Gynecologist, Surgeon. https://www.draliabadi.com/menopause/joint-pain-and-menopause/

Capel-Alcaraz, A. M., García-López, H., Castro-Sánchez, A. M., Fernández-Sánchez, M., & Lara-Palomo, I. C. (2023). "The efficacy of strength exercises for reducing the symptoms of menopause: A systematic review." *Journal of Clinical Medicine, 12(2), 548.* https://doi.org/10.3390/jcm12020548

Cramer, H., Lauche, R., Langhorst, J., & Dobos, G. (2012). "Effectiveness of yoga for menopausal symptoms: A systematic review and meta-analysis of randomized controlled trials." *Evidence-Based Complementary and Alternative Medicine: ECAM, 2012, 1–11.* https://doi.org/10.1155/2012/863905

Deeks, A. A., & McCabe, M. P. (2004). "Well-being and menopause: An investigation of purpose in life, self-acceptance and social role in premenopausal, perimenopausal and postmenopausal women." *Quality of Life Research: An International Journal of Quality of Life Aspects of Treatment, Care and Rehabilitation, 13(2), 389–398.* https://doi.org/10.1023/b:qure.0000018506.33706.05

Filipović, T. N., Lazović, M. P., Backović, A. N., Filipović, A. N., Ignjatović, A. M., Dimitrijević, S. S., & Gopčević, K. R. (2021). "A 12-week exercise program improves functional status in postmenopausal osteoporotic women: randomized controlled study." *European Journal of Physical and Rehabilitation Medicine, 57(1).* https://doi.org/10.23736/s1973-9087.20.06149-3

"Fitness." (2023, December 5). Mayo Clinic. https://www.mayoclinic.org/healthy-lifestyle/fitness/in-depth/fitness/art-20048269

Gilbert, J. (2022, September 28). "Yoga for menopause: A complete guide." *Movement for Modern Life Blog.* https://movementformodern-life.com/blog/yoga-for-menopause/

Higgins, L. (2023, June 6). "5 types of exercise that can support you during menopause." *Real Simple.* https://www.realsimple.com/exercise-for-menopause-7509018

"Joint pain." (n.d.). *My Menopause Centre.* Retrieved December 30, 2023, from https://www.mymenopausecentre.com/symptoms/joint-pain/

Ko, S.-H., & Jung, Y. (2021). "Energy metabolism changes and dysregulated lipid metabolism in postmenopausal women." *Nutrients, 13(12), 4556.* https://doi.org/10.3390/nu13124556

Mason, C., Foster-Schubert, K. E., Imayama, I., Kong, A., Xiao, L., Bain, C., Campbell, K. L., Wang, C.-Y., Duggan, C. R., Ulrich, C. M., Alfano, C. M., Blackburn, G. L., & McTiernan, A. (2011). "Dietary weight loss and exercise effects on insulin resistance in postmenopausal women." *American Journal of Preventive Medicine, 41(4), 366–375.* https://doi.org/10.1016/j.amepre.2011.06.042

"Menopause & exercise, menopause management tips." (n.d.). *Menopause.org.* Retrieved December 30, 2023, from https://www.menopause.org/for-women/menopauseflashes/exercise-and-diet/fitness-after-40-building-the-right-workout-for-a-better-body

"Menopause and the cardiovascular system." (2023, January 5). *Hopkinsmedicine.org.* https://www.hopkinsmedicine.org/health/conditions-and-diseases/menopause-and-the-cardiovascular-system

"Menopause Joint Pain: Causes & Treatment Options." (2023, February 9). *Evernow.com.* https://www.evernow.com/learn/menopause-joint-pain

"Menopause Self-esteem." (2023, November 30). *Meno Martha International Menopause Directory;* Meno Martha International Menopause Directory showcases evidence-based information by menopause societies and international sources. https://menomartha.com/health-topic/menopause-self-esteem/

"Metabolism." (n.d.). Cleveland Clinic. Retrieved December 30, 2023, from https://my.clevelandclinic.org/health/body/21893-metabolism

Mishra, N., Mishra, V. N., & Devanshi. (2011). "Exercise beyond menopause: Dos and don'ts." *Journal of Mid-Life Health, 2(2), 51.* https://doi.org/10.4103/0976-7800.92524

Moore, J. (2021, November 23). "Mental health & menopause: Why body love is so important for self esteem." MenoMe®; Meno-Me Ltd. https://www.meno-me.com/mental-health-self-esteem-menopause/

"Personal stories - Sue." (2018, October 12). *My Menopause Transformation.* https://www.mymenopausetransformation.com/personal-stories/personal-stories-sue/

"Physical activity - how to get active when you are busy." (n.d.). *Gov. au.* Retrieved December 30, 2023, from https://www.betterhealth.vic.gov.au/health/healthyliving/Physical-activity-how-to-get-active-when-you-are-busy

Riaz, H., Babur, M. N., & Farooq, A. (2022). "Effects of high-intensity multi-modal exercise training (HIT-MMEX) on bone mineral density and muscle performance in postmenopausal women. A Pilot randomized controlled trial." *JPMA. The Journal of the Pakistan Medical Association, 72(10).* https://doi.org/10.47391/jpma.5394

Sanchez, M. (2022, August 22). "Menopause weight gain: Possible causes and tips to stay healthy." *HealthPartners Blog*; HealthPartners. https://www.healthpartners.com/blog/menopause-weight-gain/

Sayer, A. (2023, August 21). "Wall Pilates guide: Try these 4 wall Pilates exercises for beginners." *Marathon Handbook.* https://marathonhandbook.com/wall-pilates/

Talks, T. [@TEDx]. (2020, June 15). "What women in menopause learned about exercise may be A lie" | Debra Atkinson | TEDxMountPenn. *Youtube.* https://www.youtube.com/watch?v=k5IzLZ1mP94

"The link between menopause and joint pain." (n.d.). *Proliance Orthopedic.* Retrieved December 30, 2023, from https://www.prolianceorthopedicassociates.com/news/the-link-between-menopause-and-joint-pain

"The reality of menopause weight gain." (2023, July 8). Mayo Clinic. https://www.mayoclinic.org/healthy-lifestyle/womens-health/in-depth/menopause-weight-gain/art-20046058

"Tips to help you exercise more, get active, NHLBI, NIH." (n.d.). *Nih. gov*. Retrieved December 30, 2023, from https://www.nhlbi.nih.gov/health/educational/wecan/get-active/getting-active.htm

West, M. (n.d.). "Mae West Quote. A-Z Quotes." Retrieved December 30, 2023, from https://www.azquotes.com/quote/365764

"Women's stories about menopause THE NEXT CHAPTER." (n.d.). *Womenfirst.com*. Retrieved December 30, 2023, from https://www.womenfirst.com/wp-content/uploads/2022/10/The_Next_Chapter_Proof-English.pdf

Chapter 4

Akan, M., Unal, S., Gonenir Erbay, L., & Taskapan, M. C. (2023). "The effect of Ramadan fasting on mental health and some hormonal levels in healthy males." *The Egyptian Journal of Neurology, Psychiatry and Neurosurgery, 59(1)*. https://doi.org/10.1186/s41983-023-00623-9

Barrea, L., Pugliese, G., Laudisio, D., Colao, A., Savastano, S., & Muscogiuri, G. (2021). "Mediterranean diet as medical prescription in menopausal women with obesity: a practical guide for nutritionists." *Critical Reviews in Food Science and Nutrition, 61(7), 1201–1211.* https://doi.org/10.1080/10408398.2020.1755220

British Heart Foundation. (2018, February 19). "Mediterranean meal tips." *British Heart Foundation.* https://www.bhf.org.uk/informationsupport/heart-matters-magazine/nutrition/mediterranean-diet/mediterranean-meal-tips

Cienfuegos, S., Corapi, S., Gabel, K., Ezpeleta, M., Kalam, F., Lin, S., Pavlou, V., & Varady, K. A. (2022). "Effect of intermittent fasting on reproductive hormone levels in females and males: A review of human trials." *Nutrients, 14(11), 2343.* https://doi.org/10.3390/nu14112343

Clinic, C. (2023, July 17). "Why intermittent fasting may be less effective for some women." Cleveland Clinic. https://health.clevelandclinic.org/intermittent-fasting-for-women/

Elsayed, M. M., Rabiee, A., El Refaye, G. E., & Elsisi, H. F. (2022). "Aerobic exercise with Mediterranean-DASH intervention for Neurodegenerative Delay diet promotes brain cells' longevity despite sex hormone deficiency in postmenopausal women: A randomized controlled trial." *Oxidative Medicine and Cellular Longevity, 2022, 1–8.* https://doi.org/10.1155/2022/4146742

"How do I start fasting? Intermittent fasting." (n.d.). *MedicineNet.* Retrieved December 30, 2023, from https://www.medicinenet.com/how_do_i_start_fasting/article.htm

"Intermittent Fasting: What is it, and how does it work?" (2023, September 29). *Hopkinsmedicine.org.* https://www.hopkinsmedicine.org/health/wellness-and-prevention/intermittent-fasting-what-is-it-and-how-does-it-work

Leonard, J. (2023, February 3). *Intermittent Fasting: Seven Ways to do Intermittent Fasting.*

"Mediterranean diet for heart health." (2023, July 15). Mayo Clinic. https://www.mayoclinic.org/healthy-lifestyle/nutrition-and-healthy-eating/in-depth/mediterranean-diet/art-20047801

Migala, J., & Kayli Anderson, R. D. N. (n.d.). "7 types of intermittent fasting: Which is best for you?" *Everydayhealth.com.* Retrieved December 30, 2023, from https://www.everydayhealth.com/diet-nutrition/diet/types-intermittent-fasting-which-best-you/

University of Illinois Chicago. (2022, October 25). "How intermittent fasting affects female hormones." *Science Daily.* https://www.science-daily.com/releases/2022/10/221025150257.htm

Vetrani, C., Barrea, L., Rispoli, R., Verde, L., De Alteriis, G., Docimo, A., Auriemma, R. S., Colao, A., Savastano, S., & Muscogiuri, G. (2022). "Mediterranean Diet: What are the consequences for menopause?" *Frontiers in Endocrinology, 13.* https://doi.org/10.3389/fendo.2022.886824

Chapter 5

Alateeq, K., Walsh, E. I., & Cherbuin, N. (2023). "Dietary magnesium intake is related to larger brain volumes and lower white matter lesions with notable sex differences." *European Journal of Nutrition, 62(5), 2039–2051.* https://doi.org/10.1007/s00394-023-03123-x

Hersh, E. (2020, August 17). "Sleep hygiene explained and 10 tips for better sleep." *Healthline.* https://www.healthline.com/health/sleep-hygiene

Herstasis Health [@herstasishealth]. (2023, January 26). "Surviving breast cancer and the aftermath of medically-induced menopause." *Youtube.* https://www.youtube.com/watch?v=NEK32ceCjto

"How to fall asleep faster and sleep better." (n.d.). *Nhs.uk.* Retrieved December 30, 2023, from https://www.nhs.uk/every-mind-matters/mental-wellbeing-tips/how-to-fall-asleep-faster-and-sleep-better/

Kalmbach, D. A., Cheng, P., Arnedt, J. T., Anderson, J. R., Roth, T., Fellman-Couture, C., Williams, R. A., & Drake, C. L. (2019). "Treating insomnia improves depression, maladaptive thinking, and hyperarousal in postmenopausal women: comparing cognitive-behavioral therapy for insomnia (CBTI), sleep restriction therapy, and sleep hygiene education." *Sleep Medicine, 55, 124–134.* https://doi.org/10.1016/j.sleep.2018.11.019

Losso, J. N., Finley, J. W., Karki, N., Liu, A. G., Prudente, A., Tipton, R., Yu, Y., & Greenway, F. L. (2018). "Pilot study of the tart cherry juice for the treatment of insomnia and investigation of mechanisms." *American Journal of Therapeutics, 25(2), e194–e201.* https://doi.org/10.1097/mjt.0000000000000584

"Pins and needles." (n.d.). *Nhs.uk.* Retrieved December 30, 2023, from https://www.nhs.uk/conditions/pins-and-needles/

"Restless legs syndrome." (n.d.). *Nhs.uk.* Retrieved December 30, 2023, from https://www.nhs.uk/conditions/restless-legs-syndrome/

"Sleep and menopause." (n.d.). *WebMD*. Retrieved December 30, 2023, from https://www.webmd.com/menopause/sleep-disorders-sleep-menopause

Summer, J. (2009, April 17). "Napping: Benefits and tips | sleep foundation." *Sleep Foundation*.

Suni, E. (2009, April 17). "Mastering sleep hygiene: Your path to quality sleep | sleep foundation." *Sleep Foundation*.

"The best and worst foods for sleep." (2020, October 15). *Benenden Health*. https://www.benenden.co.uk/be-healthy/nutrition/the-best-and-worst-foods-for-sleep/

TODAY [@TODAY]. (2018, August 31). "Mother takes action after battling insomnia for 4 years: 'I just want to sleep' | Megyn Kelly TODAY." *Youtube*. https://www.youtube.com/watch?v=Km6Unhybhsg

Vázquez-Lorente, H., Herrera-Quintana, L., Molina-López, J., Gamarra-Morales, Y., López-González, B., Miralles-Adell, C., & Planells, E. (2020). "Response of vitamin D after magnesium intervention in a postmenopausal population from the province of Granada, Spain." *Nutrients, 12(8), 2283*. https://doi.org/10.3390/nu12082283

Wesström, J., Nilsson, S., Sundström-Poromaa, I., & Ulfberg, J. (2008). "Restless legs syndrome among women: prevalence, co-morbidity and possible relationship to menopause." *Climacteric: The Journal of the International Menopause Society, 11(5), 422–428*. https://doi.org/10.1080/13697130802359683

Chapter 6

"10 ways to create an emotionally healthy home." (n.d.). *Psychology Today*. Retrieved December 30, 2023, from https://www.psychologytoday.com/intl/blog/what-mentally-strong-people-dont-do/202009/10-ways-create-emotionally-healthy-home

Daly, H. (2023, July 18). "How to talk to your family about the menopause." *My Menopause Centre.* https://www.mymenopausecentre.com/blog/how-to-talk-about-the-menopause/

Elizabeth, D. (2022, October 19). "45 loving affirmations for menopause." *Wild Simple Joy.* https://wildsimplejoy.com/loving-affirmations-for-menopause/

"Emotional wellness toolkit." (2017, April 7). *National Institutes of Health (NIH).* https://www.nih.gov/health-information/emotional-wellness-toolkit

Gillihan, S. (n.d.). "10 ways to boost your emotional health." *Everydayhealth.com.* Retrieved December 30, 2023, from https://www.everydayhealth.com/emotional-health/10-ways-to-boost-emotional-health.aspx

Godden, J. (2021, January 28). "Anxiety, menopause, and the power of mindfulness." *Stella*; Vira Health. https://www.onstella.com/the-latest/anxiety-and-mood/how-mindfulness-can-help-ease-anxiety/

Gordon, J. L., Halleran, M., Beshai, S., Eisenlohr-Moul, T. A., Frederick, J., & Campbell, T. S. (2021). "Endocrine and psychosocial moderators of mindfulness-based stress reduction for the prevention of perimenopausal depressive symptoms: A randomized controlled trial." *Psychoneuroendocrinology, 130(105277), 105277.* https://doi.org/10.1016/j.psyneuen.2021.105277

horm. (2018, December 10). "10 ways to combat menopause mood swings." *Hormone Health.* https://hormonehealth.co.uk/10-ways-to-even-out-your-menopause-mood-swings

Julia, H. (2020, February 3). "The benefits and importance of a support system." *Highland Springs.* https://highlandspringsclinic.org/the-benefits-and-importance-of-a-support-system/

Kapil, R. (2020, August 6). "The importance of having a support system." *Mental Health First Aid.* https://www.mentalhealthfirstaid.org/2020/08/the-importance-of-having-a-support-system/

Killoran, E. (2013, November 11). "The menopause years and beyond." *Pritikin Luxury Wellness Retreat.* https://www.pritikin.com/your-health/ healthy-living/womens-health/136-17-lifestyle-tips-for-the-meno-pause-years-and-beyond.html

"Lifestyle changes for menopause." (n.d.). *Nyulangone.org.* Retrieved December 30, 2023, from https://nyulangone.org/conditions/menopause/ treatments/lifestyle-changes-for-menopause

"Menopause Mood Swings." (n.d.). *Sutterhealth.org.* Retrieved December 30, 2023, from https://www.sutterhealth.org/health/womens-health/ menopause-mood-swings

Seo, R. D. (n.d.). "Talking about menopause with friends and family." *Com.au.* Retrieved December 30, 2023, from https://www.menopause-centre.com.au/information-centre/articles/talking-about-menopause-with-friends-and-family/

Vogel UK, A. [@AvogelCoUk]. (2022, August 1). "Perimenopause rage: what causes it & how to manage it." *Youtube.* https://www.youtube.com/ watch?v=uJ4Tni84USc

Chapter 7

"Decreased Desire." (n.d.). *Menopause.org.* Retrieved December 30, 2023, from https://www.menopause.org/for-women/sexual-health-menopause-online/ sexual-problems-at-midlife/decreased-desire

Dording, C. M., Schettler, P. J., Dalton, E. D., Parkin, S. R., Walker, R. S. W., Fehling, K. B., Fava, M., & Mischoulon, D. (2015). "A double-blind placebo-controlled trial of maca root as treatment for anti-depressant-induced sexual dysfunction in women." *Evidence-Based Complementary and Alternative Medicine: ECAM, 2015, 1–9.* https://doi. org/10.1155/2015/949036

Goldwert, L. (2022, October 24). "Menopause and sex: How to keep things sexy with your partner." *Stripes.* https://iamstripes.com/blogs/ sex-sex-sex/keeping-things-sexy-with-your-partner-during-menopause

Hersh, E. (2017, May 9). "Menopause and libido: Does menopause affect sex drive?" *Healthline*. https://www.healthline.com/health/menopause/menopause-libido

"How to have great sex during menopause and beyond." (2021, May 14). *Nebraskamed.com*. https://www.nebraskamed.com/womens-health/how-to-have-great-sex-during-menopause

Junggren, M. (2021, July 14). "How to talk about sex with your partner during menopause." *Bonafide*. https://hellobonafide.com/blogs/news/how-to-talk-about-sex-with-your-partner-during-menopause

"Low libido during middle age: How to spice up your sex life." (n.d.). *Inspiriko*. Retrieved December 30, 2023, from https://inspiriko.co.uk/blogs/article/low-libido-during-middle-age-how-to-spice-up-your-sex-life

People, O. (n.d.). "Can menopause cause relationship breakdown?" *Crisp and Co.* Retrieved December 30, 2023, from https://www.crispandco.com/site/blog/family-law-blog/can-menopause-cause-relationship-breakdown

Pycroft, L. (2021, July 1). "Building emotional and sexual intimacy during menopause." *Stella*; Vira Health. https://www.onstella.com/the-latest/sex-and-relationships/building-a-bridge-to-emotional-and-sexual-intimacy/

"Relationship Issues." (n.d.). *Menopause.org*. Retrieved December 30, 2023, from https://www.menopause.org/for-women/sexual-health-menopause-online/causes-of-sexual-problems/relationship-issues

"Sex and menopause." (n.d.). *WebMD*. Retrieved December 30, 2023, from https://www.webmd.com/menopause/sex-menopause

"Sexual wellbeing, intimacy and menopause." (2023, March 14). *NHS Inform*. https://www.nhsinform.scot/healthy-living/womens-health/later-years-around-50-years-and-over/menopause-and-post-menopause-health/sexual-wellbeing-intimacy-and-menopause/

Thomas, H. N., Brotto, L. A., de Abril Cameron, F., Yabes, J., & Thurston, R. C. (2023). "A virtual, group-based mindfulness intervention for midlife and older women with low libido lowers sexual distress in a randomized controlled pilot study." *The Journal of Sexual Medicine, 20(8), 1060–1068.* https://doi.org/10.1093/jsxmed/qdad081

Chapter 8

"11 supplements for menopause." (n.d.). *WebMD.* Retrieved December 30, 2023, from https://www.webmd.com/menopause/ss/slideshow-menopause

"Better skin after menopause." (n.d.). *WebMD.* Retrieved December 30, 2023, from https://www.webmd.com/menopause/ss/slideshow-better-skin-after-menopause

Beverton, D. (2022, February 16). "Menopause clothing: How to look good and have fun." *Stella*; Vira Health. https://www.onstella.com/the-latest/her-story/how-to-look-good-during-menopause-and-have-fun/

Blum, K. (2023, May 24). "Should you prescribe bioidentical hormones for menopause?" *Medscape.* https://www.medscape.com/viewarticle/992412?form=fpf

Bringle, J. (2021, May 27). "When I couldn't find relief, needles helped my menopause symptoms." *Healthline.* https://www.healthline.com/health/menopause/acupuncture-for-menopause-how-this-alternative-therapy-brought-me-relief

"Caring for your skin in menopause." (n.d.). *Aad.org.* Retrieved December 30, 2023, from https://www.aad.org/public/everyday-care/skin-care-secrets/anti-aging/skin-care-during-menopause

Clinic, C. (2021, February 19). "Here's how menopause affects your skin and hair." *Cleveland Clinic.* https://health.clevelandclinic.org/heres-how-menopause-affects-your-skin-and-hair/

Draelos, Z. D., Diaz, I., Namkoong, J., Wu, J., & Boyd, T. (2021). "Efficacy evaluation of a topical hyaluronic acid serum in facial photoaging." *Dermatology and Therapy, 11(4), 1385–1394.* https://doi.org/10.1007/s13555-021-00566-0

Haver, M. C. [@maryclairehavermd8473]. (2022, October 26). "What supplements I take in menopause and why." *Youtube.* https://www.youtube.com/watch?v=vs6SEITM02k

"How to dress during menopause - the best outfit tricks to complement your hot and cold body." (n.d.). *Sunday Telegraph.* Retrieved December 30, 2023, from https://www.telegraph.co.uk/fashion/style/what-wear-during-menopause-how-dress-hot-cold-body-outfits/

Juncan, A. M., Moisă, D. G., Santini, A., Morgovan, C., Rus, L.-L., Vonica-Țincu, A. L., & Loghin, F. (2021). "Advantages of hyaluronic acid and its combination with other bioactive ingredients in cosmeceuticals." *Molecules (Basel, Switzerland), 26(15), 4429.* https://doi.org/10.3390/molecules26154429

kellis. (2022, July 31). "Dressing through and beyond the menopause." Image Consultant & Personal Stylist; Kerrie Ellis - Image Consultant. https://www.kerrieellis.co.uk/2022/07/31/dressing-through-and-beyond-the-menopause/

Luong, R. (2023, May 1). "Stacy London's 6 styling tips for menopausal women + viewer gets ultimate makeover." *Rachael Ray Show.* https://www.rachaelrayshow.com/articles/stacy-londons-6-styling-tips-for-menopausal-women-viewer-gets-ultimate-makeover

Mayer, B. A. (2022, September 1). "Derms share top tips to care for your skin in menopause." *Healthline.* https://www.healthline.com/health/beauty-skin-care/dermatologists-share-skin-care-tips-for-menopause-and-beyond

"Menopause supplements: 10 best vitamins to manage symptoms." (n.d.). *Gennev.com.* Retrieved December 30, 2023, from https://www.gennev.com/education/vitamins-for-menopause-symptoms

Milani, M., & Sparavigna, A. (2017). "The 24-hour skin hydration and barrier function effects of a hyaluronic 1%, glycerin 5%, and Centella asiatica stem cells extract moisturizing fluid: an intra-subject, randomized, assessor-blinded study." *Clinical, Cosmetic and Investigational Dermatology, 10, 311–315.* https://doi.org/10.2147/ccid.s144180

Olvera, L. (2022, July 20). "Hair and skin changes: perimenopause and menopause." *Clue.* https://helloclue.com/articles/skin-and-hair/hair-and-skin-changes-perimenopause-and-menopause

Seo, R. D. (n.d.). "The benefits of acupuncture for reducing menopausal symptoms." *Com.au.* Retrieved December 30, 2023, from https://www.menopausecentre.com.au/information-centre/articles/acupuncture-reducing-menopausal-symptoms/

Shaw, S. (2022, December 12). "What is menopausal skin care? Experts explain the benefits and share the 17 best products." CNN. https://www.cnn.com/cnn-underscored/beauty/menopause-skincare-guide

Simmonds, L. (2022, January 23). "Style tips for menopausal women." *The Fearless Fashionista.*https://thefearlessfashionista.com/blog/style-tips-4-menopausal-women-2zdhx

"Skin disorders during menopause." (2016, February 12). *Mdedge. com*; Frontline Medical Communications Inc. https://www.mdedge.com/dermatology/article/106506/aesthetic-dermatology/skin-disorders-during-menopause

Spada, F., Barnes, T. M., & Greive, K. A. (2018). "Skin hydration is significantly increased by a cream formulated to mimic the skin's own natural moisturizing systems." *Clinical, Cosmetic and Investigational Dermatology, 11, 491–497.* https://doi.org/10.2147/ccid.s177697

"Turmeric & menopause relief." (n.d.). *The 'Pause Life by Dr. Mary Claire Haver.* Retrieved December 30, 2023, from https://galvestondiet.com/nutritional-supplements/turmeric-menopause-relief/

"What is Menopausal Hormone Therapy (MHT) and is it safe?" (n.d.). *Org.au.* Retrieved January 1, 2024, from https://www.menopause.org.au/health-info/fact-sheets/what-is-menopausal-hormone-therapy-mht-and-is-it-safe

"What to wear during menopause - 6 tips to feel & look your best." (2023, May 2). *Busbee - Fashion Over 40.* https://busbeestyle.com/what-to-wear-during-menopause/

Williams, F. (2022, April 14). "10 ways to style your way through menopause and increase body confidence." *Rest Less.* https://restless.co.uk/leisure-and-lifestyle/home-garden/ways-to-style-your-way-through-menopause-and-increase-body-confidence/

Younkin, L. (2023, June 8). "The 7 best supplements for menopause, according to a dietitian." *Verywell Health.* https://www.verywellhealth.com/best-supplements-for-menopause-7505896

Zouboulis, C. C., Blume-Peytavi, U., Kosmadaki, M., Roó, E., Vexiau-Robert, D., Kerob, D., & Goldstein, S. R. (2022). "Skin, hair and beyond: the impact of menopause." *Climacteric: The Journal of the International Menopause Society, 25(5), 434–442.* https://doi.org/10.1080/13697137.2022.2050206

www.ingramcontent.com/pod-product-compliance
Lightning Source LLC
Chambersburg PA
CBHW052019030426
42335CB00026B/3203